ᓂᕆᔭᒃᓴᐃᑦ ᐃᓅᓕᓴᐅᑎᐅᓃᑦ
ᐅᑭᐅᖅᑕᖅᑐᒥ ᐱᕈ
ᐃᓅᑉ ᐃᓐᓇᐅᑉ ᑕᑯ

Edible and Medicinal Arctic Plants

An Inuit Elder's Perspective

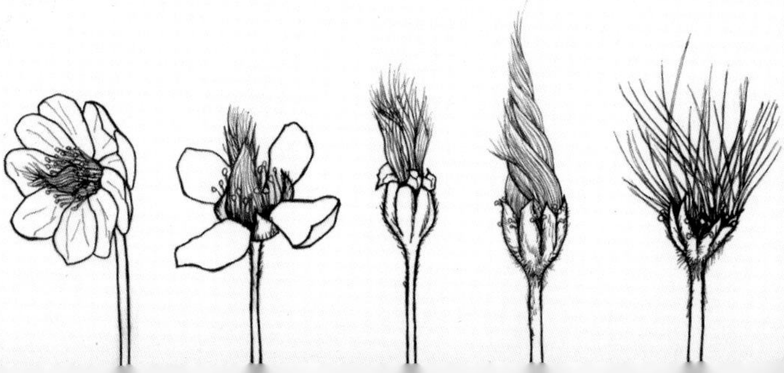

Published by Inhabit Media Inc. | www.inhabitmedia.com

Inhabit Media Inc. (Iqaluit), P.O. Box 11125, Iqaluit, Nunavut, X0A 1H0
(Toronto), 191 Eglinton Avenue East, Suite 301, Toronto, Ontario, M4P 1K1

First edition published 2009. Second edition 2018.

Edited by Neil Christopher
Translated by Rebecca Hainnu and Louise Flaherty
Researched by Aalasi Joamie, Anna Ziegler, and Rebecca Hainnu
Art direction by Danny Christopher
Cover design by Astrid Arijanto
Photography by Anna Ziegler (except where noted)

Published by Inhabit Media in collaboration with the Nunavut Bilingual Education Society with funding from the Department of Culture and Heritage. Text in English and Inuktitut.

We acknowledge the support of the Canada Council for the Arts for our publishing program.

This project was made possible in part by the Government of Canada.

ISBN: 978-1-77227-170-6

Library and Archives Canada Cataloguing in Publication

Ziegler, Anna, 1979-, author
Ukiuqtaqtumi piruqtut nirijaksait inuulisautiusuullu : inuup innaup takkuanit / Ana Siiglur, Alasi Juumi, Riipika Hainnu = Edible and medicinal Arctic plants : an Inuit elder's perspective / Anna Ziegler, Aalasi Joamie, Rebecca Hainnu.

Revision of: Walking with Aalasi.
Text in Inuktitut syllabics and English. Title romanized.
ISBN 978-1-77227-170-6 (softcover)

1. Plants, Edible--Nunavut. 2. Medicinal plants--Nunavut. 3. Traditional ecological knowledge--Nunavut. I. Joamie, Aalasi, author II. Hainnu, Rebecca, author III. Ziegler, Anna, 1979- . Walking with Aalasi. IV. Ziegler, Anna, 1979- . Walking with Aalasi. Inuktitut. V. Title. VI. Title: Edible and medicinal Arctic plants.

SB294.C3Z54 2018 581.6'34097195 C2017-907824-0

Printed in Canada

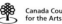

INHABIT MEDIA
NBES
Nunavut
Canadian Heritage Patrimoine canadien
Canada Council for the Arts Conseil des Arts du Canada
Canada

ᓂᕆᔭᒃᓴᐃᑦ ᐃᓅᓯᓕᓴᐅᑎᐅᓲᑦᓗ ᐅᑭᐅᖅᑕᖅᑐᒥ ᐱᕈᖅᑐᑦ

ᐃᓅᑉ ᐃᓐᓇᐅᑉ ᑕᒃᑯᐊᓂᑦ

Edible and Medicinal Arctic Plants

An Inuit Elder's Perspective

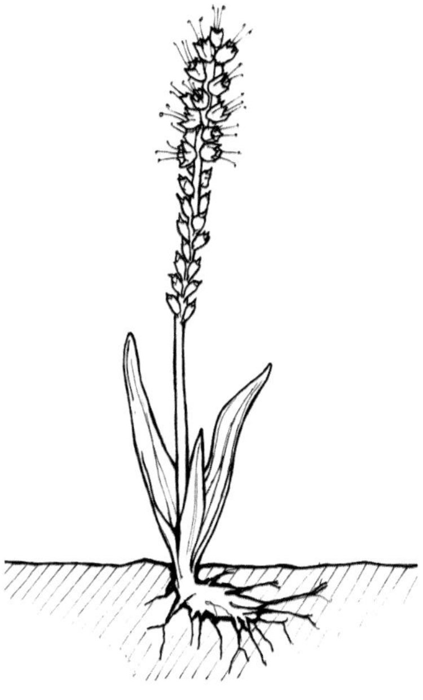

ᐋᓇ ᓰᒡᓗᕐ
Anna Ziegler

ᐋᓚᓯ ᔫᒥ
Aalasi Joamie

ᕇᐱᑲ ᕼᐊᐃᓐᓄ
Rebecca Hainnu

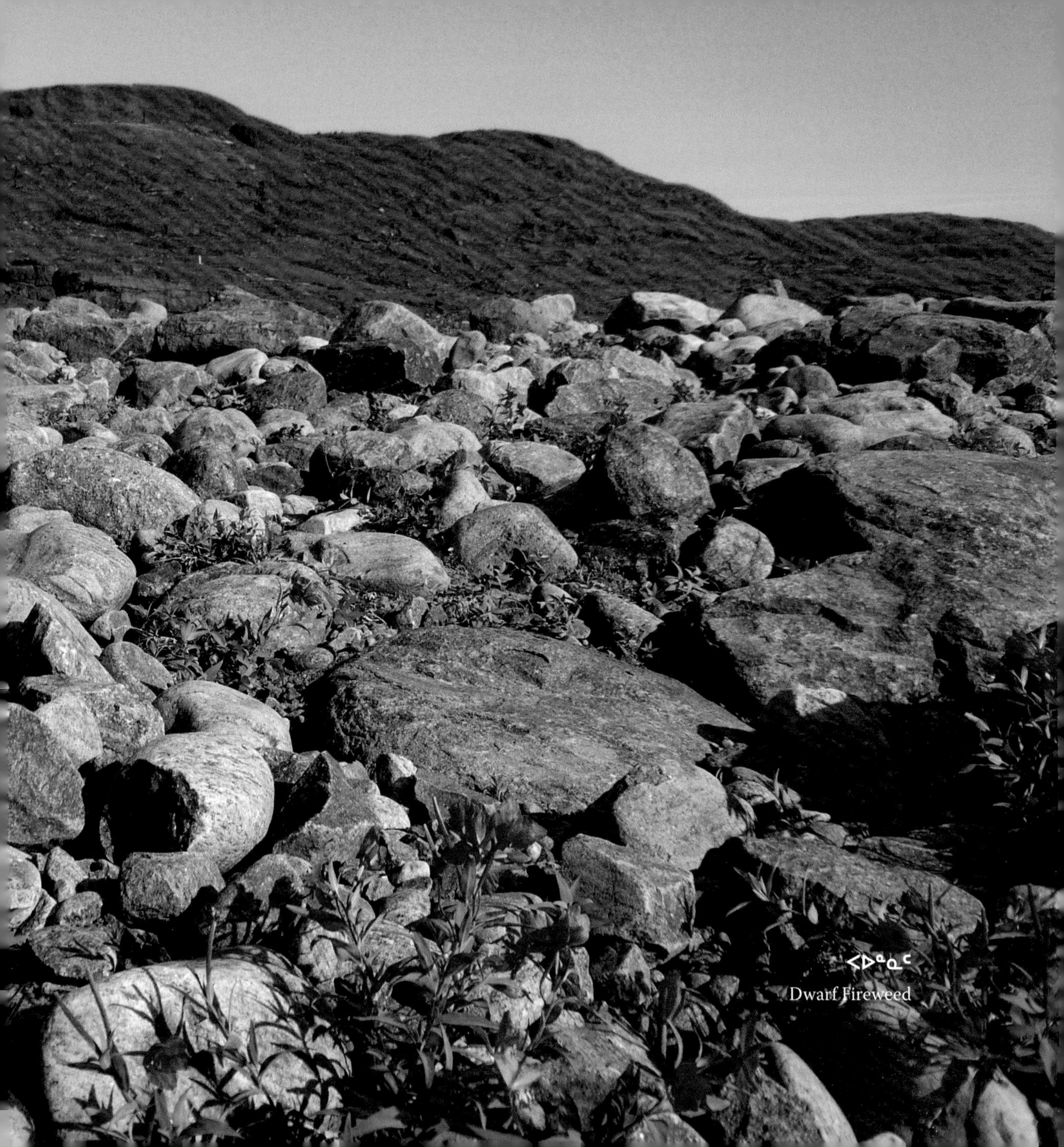

ᐸᐅᓐᓇᑦ

Dwarf Fireweed

ᐃᓗᓕᖏᑦ
Table of Contents

ᐅᖃᓕᒫᒐᐅᑉ ᒥᒃᓵᓄᑦ ᐅᖃᐅᓯᒃᓴᑦ
Preface 1

ᖁᔭᓐᓇᒦᖅᑕᐅᔪᑦ
Acknowledgements 3

ᐱᓕᕆᐊᑦ ᒥᒃᓵᓄᑦ
About This Project 5

ᑕᑯᑎᑦᑎᒥᐊᕈᑎ ᐋᓚᓯ ᔫᒥᒦᖖᒑᖅᑐᑦ
Introduction by Aalasi Joamie 8

ᓇᓗᓇᐃᒃᑯᑕᑦ ᐱᕈᖅᑑᑉ ᐊᑑᑎᖏᓐᓄᑦ ᐊᑎᖏᓐᓄᓗ
Summary of Plant Uses and Names 17

ᐱᕈᖅᑐᑦ
Plants 21

ᐳᐊᓗᖖᒍᐊᑦ
Pualunnguat / Arctic Cotton 23

ᒪᓂᖅ
Maniq / Lamp Moss. 29

ᐅᖅᐱ ᓱᐳᑎᓪᓗ
Uqpi Suputillu / Arctic Willow 33

ᖁᐊᕋᐃᑦ
Quarait / Snow-Bed Willow. 39

ᐊᓚᒃᓴᐅᔭᐃᑦ
Alaksaujait / Net-Vein Willow 43

ᐸᐅᓐᓇᐃᑦ
Paunnait / Dwarf Fireweed 47

ᖁᖑᓖᑦ
Qunguliit / Mountain Sorrel 55

ᓴᐸᖓᕋᓛᙳᐊᑦ ᑐᖅᑕᐃᓪᓗ
Sapangaralaannguat Tuqtaillu / Alpine Bistort 61

ᐸᐅᕐᖓᐃᑦ ᐊᔾᔨᒌᖏᑦᑐᑦ
Paurngait Ajjigiingittut / Berry Plants 67

ᐸᐅᕐᖓᐃᑦ ᐸᐅᕐᖓᖁᑎᓪᓗ
Paurngait Paurngaqutillu / Crowberry 68

ᑲᓪᓚᐃᑦ ᑲᓪᓚᖁᑎᓪᓗ
Kallait Kallaqutillu / Bearberry 72

ᑭᒍᑕᖏᕐᓇᐃᑦ ᓇᖁᑎᓪᓗ
Kigutangirnait Naqutillu / Blueberry 75

ᐸᐅᕐᖓᓂᑦ ᐊᑐᕐᓂᐊᕐᓗᓂ
Using Berry Plants 78

ᕿᔪᒃᑖᖅᐸᐃᑦ
Qijuktaaqpait / Labrador Tea 81

ᓯᐅᕋᐅᑉ ᐅᖃᐅᔭᖏᑦ
Siuraup Uqaujangit / Seaside Bluebells 87

ᒪᓕᒃᑳᑦ
Malikkaat / Mountain Avens 93

ᐅᕐᔪ
Urju / Peat Moss 99

ᐃᔾᓯᐅᑎ
Ijisiuti / River Algae 105

ᓂᕐᓇᐃᑦ
Nirnait / Snow Lichen 109

ᐳᔪᐊᓗᒃ
Pujualuk / Dried Mushroom 113

ᐊᑐᒐᒃᓴᒃᑲᓐᓃᑦ
Additional Resources 116

ᑎᑎᕋᖅᑐᕕᓃᑦ
Contributors 118

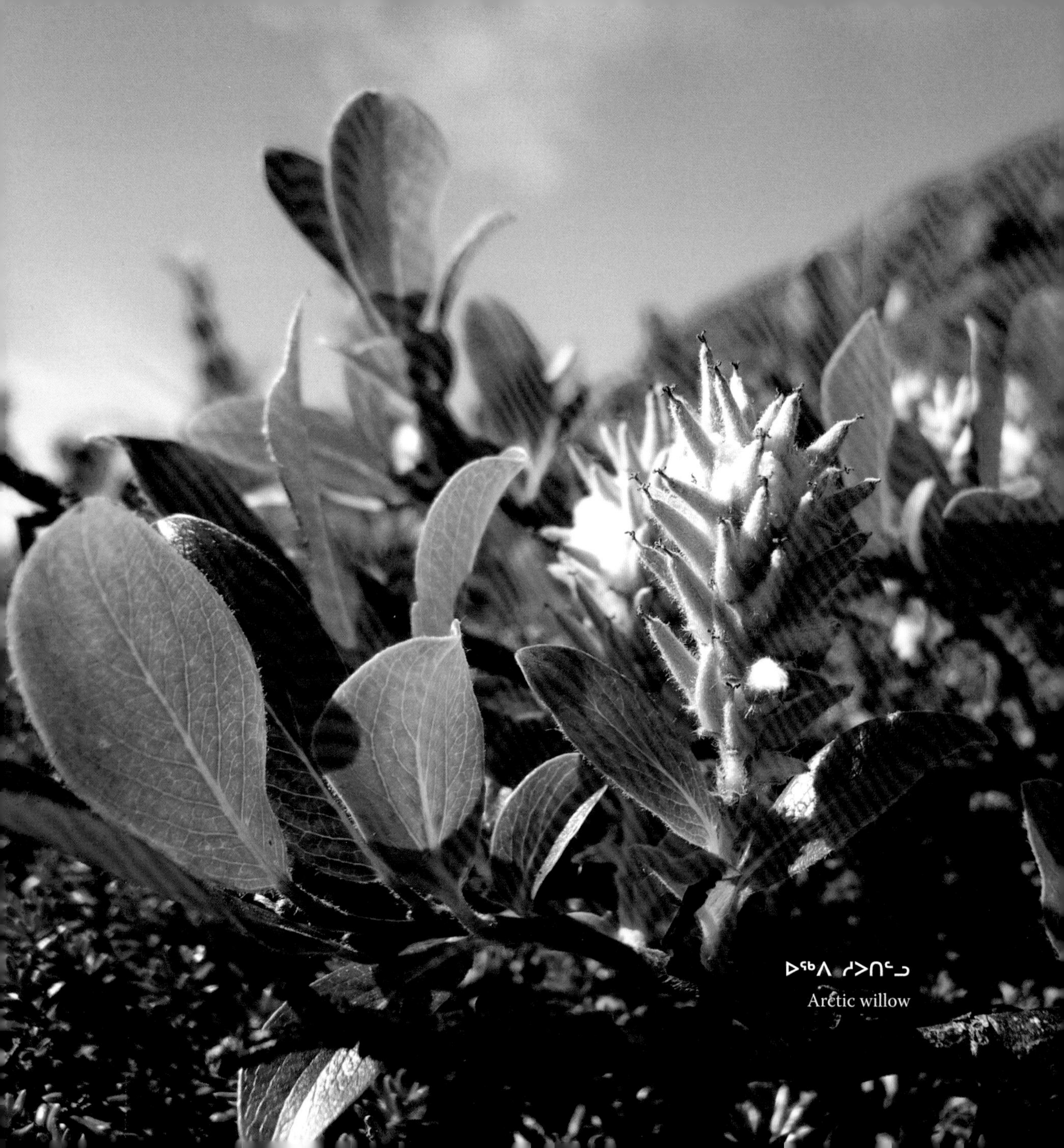

ᐅᖅᐱ ᓱᐳᑎᑦᓗ

Arctic willow

ᐅᖃᓕᒫᒐᐅᑉ ᒥᒃᓵᓄᑦ ᐅᖃᐅᓯᒃᓴᑦ

Preface

ᐊᕐᕌᒍᑦ ᖁᓕᐅᐸᔫᓕᖅᑐᑦ ᓴᖅᑭᑕᐅᓚᐅᖅᓯᒪᑎᑦᑐᒍ ᐱᓱᒃᑎᒃᑲᓂᖅ ᐋᓚᓯᒥᒃ, ᖁᕕᐊᒋᑦᑎᐊᕆᕙᕋᑦᑕᐅᖅ ᐊᒥᓱᓄᑦ ᓄᓇᕐᔪᐊᕐᒥᐅᓄᑦ ᑐᓴᕐᓂᕆᔭᐅᕙᓪᓕᒻᒪᑦ. ᑕᐃᒪᙵᓂᑦ ᐊᒥᓱᓄᑦ ᐊᐃᖃᑦᑕᖅᓯᒪᕗᖓ ᐅᖃᓕᒫᒐᓕᐅᓚᐅᖅᑎᑦᑐᖓ, ᓄᓇᓕᖕᓂ ᓱᕙᖃᓕᖐᖏᑦ, ᑲᑎᒪᔪᓄᑦ, ᖃᓄᐃᓕᐅᕈᔫᔭᖅᑐᖅᑲᖅᑎᑦᑐᒍᑐ ᐃᓕᓐᓂᐊᖅᑎᑦᑎᓯᓐᓈᑦ, ᐊᓯᖏᓐᓄᑦᑐ, ᓂᒋᕐᒦᙳᖅᓯᒪᔭᓄᑦ ᐳᓖᕆᐊᖅᑐᓄᑦ. ᑯᐄᑦᑐ ᐃᕐᓂᖓ ᑲᑎᖅᑲᑎᒋᓚᐅᕆᑦᑐᒍ ᓵᓕ ᑕᒪᐅᙳᕐᒪᑦ 2017-ᒥᑦ. ᖁᔭᓕᓚᐅᖅᑐᖅ ᐊᑐᖁᑦᓴᑦᑎᐊᕙᐅᓱᓇᑦᑐᓂᐅᑦᑐ.

It has been almost ten years since *Walking with Aalasi* was first published, and I am excited that other people around the world have enjoyed the book. It has given me a lot of opportunities since being published: being a part of community events, meetings, certain functions while educating those, others, southerners, who have come to visit. I even met the Queen's son, Prince Charles, when he was here in 2017. He was very thankful and thought it was a great resource.

ᐅᖃᓕᒫᒐᖅ ᐅᓇ ᐱᒋᐊᕈᑎᑐᐃᓐᓇᐅᕗᖅ, ᐊᒥᓱᒃᑲᓐᓂᕐᓂᒃ ᐅᖃᓕᒫᒐᖅᑖᕆᐊᖅᑲᖅᐳᒍᑦ, ᑭᖑᕚᕆᓂᐊᖅᑕᕗᑦ ᐊᓯᐅᔨᓂᐊᖏᓪᓚᑕ ᓄᓇᐅᑉ ᒥᔅᓵᓄᑦ ᖃᐅᔨᒪᓂᕐᒥᒃ. ᐊᒥᓱᓂᒃ ᐊᓯᖏᓐᓂᒃ ᐱᕈᖅᑐᖅᑕᖅᑲᐅᕐᒪᑦ ᐊᑐᕈᓐᓇᖅᑕᑦᑎᓐᓂᒃ ᐃᓅᓕᓴᐅᑎᒋᓗᑎᒍ ᓂᕆᔭᔅᓴᐅᑦᑐᑎᑦᑐ. ᐊᓯᖏᓂᑦᑐ ᐱᕈᖅᑐᖅᑕᖅᑲᐅᓇᒐᖅ ᐅᕙᑎᓐᓄᑦ ᐱᐅᖏᑦᑐᓂᒃ. ᐅᖃᓕᒫᒐᒃᑲᓐᓂᖅ ᑕᒪᔅᓱᒥ ᑐᓴᖅᑕᐅᑎᑦᑎᔪᓐᓇᖅᑲᔭᕈᕗᖅ. ᐃᓐᓇᑐᖅᑲᐳᑕᕋᒪ --ᑕᒫᓅᖏᓐᓇᔾᔪᖏᓐᓇᒪ ᖃᐅᔨᒪᓂᕋ ᑐᓴᖅᑕᐅᑎᑦᑐᒍ. ᑐᓴᖅᑕᐅᔭᕆᐊᑖᑦ ᐊᒥᓱᐊᓘᒻᒪᑕ ᐃᓅᓕᓴᐅᑏᑦ, ᓂᕿᑦ, ᑎᒥᑦᑎᓐᓄᑦᑐ ᐋᑐᑎᖅᑲᑦᑎᐊᖅᑐᑦ ᐱᕈᖅᑐᓃᙳᖅᑐᑦ ᓱᓕ ᐃᑲᔪᕈᒪᕗᖓ ᐅᖃᓕᒫᒐᓕᐅᖅᑐᖅᑲᖅᑎᑦᑐᒍ ᓯᕗᓂᒃᓴᑦᑎᓐᓂ. ᐱᕈᖅᑐᑦ ᐊᒥᓲᒻᒪᑕ ᑕᖅᑳᓂ ᐋᑐᑎᑖᑦ.

This book is a start, but I think that we need more books, to ensure that future generations do not lose this knowledge of the land. There are many other plants and flowers that can be used medicinally and to eat. There are also other plants and vegetation that are bad for us. Another book would help capture this knowledge. I'm getting old—I won't be around forever to share my knowledge. There is so much more information about medication, food, and nourishment from plants that I would love to contribute to future books. There are so many plants out there that are beneficial.

ᐊᑲᐅᓯᕙᓐᓇᖁᑦᑕᓗ ᑎᒥᕗᑦᑐ ᓴᓗᒻᒪᖅᑎᑦᑐᒍ ᓂᕆᕙᑦᑐᑕ ᐱᕈᖅᑐᓂ ᐊᕙᑎᑦᑎᓐᓃᑐᓂᒃ. ᐃᓅᓯᑦᑎᓐᓄᑦ ᐱᐅᒻᒪᑕ. ᒫᓐᓇᒃᑯᑦ ᑐᓴᖅᑲᑦᑕᓕᖁᑦᑕ ᐊᑲᐅᙱᓕᐅᕈᑎᓕᓐᓂᒃ, ᐱᓗᐊᖅᑐᓂ ᐳᕙᖕᒥᒍᑦ. ᑭᓯᐊᓂᓕ ᐃᓅᓕᓴᐅᑎᑕᖅᑲᐅᖅᐳᖅ ᑕᖅᑳᓂ ᐃᑲᔪᕈᓐᓇᖅᑐᓂᒃ.

We can heal and cleanse our bodies by eating the plants around us. They are great for our health. We are finding more and more health problems these days, especially respiratory problems with our lungs. Yet we have the medicine right outside that can help.

ᑕᐃᒃᑯᓄᖓ ᑲᙵᖅᓯᐃᖅᑲᑦᑕᕈᒪᔪᓄᑦ ᐱᕈᖅᑐᓂᒃ, ᐊᑐᐃᓐᓇᐅᑦᑎᐊᖅᑐᖓ. ᐃᑲᔪᕈᓐᓇᑦᑎᐊᖅᑐᖓ ᐃᓕᑦᑐᒪᔪᓂᒃ, ᐱᓱᖅᑲᑎᖅᑲᕈᒪᔪᓂᒃ ᐅᕙᖕᓂᑦ, ᑐᓴᒃᑲᓐᓂᕈᒪᑉᐸᑕ, ᑭᓱᑦ ᐱᐅᒻᒪᖔᑕ ᐱᐅᖏᒻᒪᖔᑕᓗ. ᓂᕆᔭᓐᓇᖅᑐᒍᑦ, ᐃᓕᓐᓂᐊᖅᑎᑦᑐᓐᓇᖅᑕᒃᑲ.

For those wanting to start harvesting their own plants, I am always available. I can help anyone who wants to learn more, who wants me to go for a walk with them, if they want more information, to tell them what is good or bad. We can eat, and I can teach them.

—ᐋᓚᓯ ᔫᒥ
ᓂᐊᖁᙳᖅ, ᓄᓇᕗᑦ, 2017

—Aalasi Joamie
Niaqunnguuq (Apex), Nunavut, 2017

ᖁᔭᓐᓇᒦᖅᑕᐅᔪᑦ
Acknowledgements

ᖁᔭᓐᓇᒦᕈᒪᔭᕗᑦ ᐃᑲᔪᖅᑲᑦᑕᓚᐅᖅᑐᑦ ᑲᔪᖕᒋᖅᓴᐃᖅᑲᑦᑕᓚᐅᖅᑐᑦᓗ ᐅᖅᑲᓕᒫᒐᖅ ᐱᔭᕇᖁᑦᑐᒍ.

We would like to acknowledge the contributions and support of the many people who helped us finish this book.

ᐋᓚᓯ ᖁᔭᓐᓇᒦᖅᑐᖅ ᐊᓈᓇᒥᓂ ᐱᕈᖅᑐᑦ ᒥᒃᓵᓂᑦ ᐃᓕᓐᓂᐊᖅᑎᑦᑎᖅᑲᑦᑕᓚᐅᕐᒪᑦ. ᐃᓕᓐᓂᐊᖅᑎᑦᑎᖅᑲᑦᑕᓚᐅᖕᒋᑉᐸᑦ ᐊᔪᕆᖅᓲᔾᔨᑐᓂᒎᓐᓂᑦ ᐋᓚᓯ ᑐᓴᐅᒪᒐᔭᓚᐅᖕᒋᓪᒪᑦ ᐅᑦᓗᒥ ᐃᓕᓐᓂᐊᖅᑎᑦᑎᔾᔪᑎᒋᖅᑲᑦᑕᓕᖅᑕᒥᓂᑦ. ᐋᓚᓯᑦᑕᐅ ᖁᔭᓐᓇᒦᕈᒪᔪᖅ ᐸᓂᑯᓗᒻᒥᓄᑦ ᔫᐋᓂᒧᑦ ᐅᖅᑲᓕᒫᒐᖅ ᓴᓇᔭᐅᕙᑦᓕᐊᑎᑦᑐᒍ ᒥᖅᓱᖅᑎᑦᑎᑎᑦᑐᒍᓘᓐᓃᑦ ᑑᓴᔨᐅᖕᒋᓐᓇᖅᑲᑦᑕᓚᐅᕐᒪᑦ.

Aalasi is grateful to her mother for teaching her about plants. Without her mother's dedicated teaching and encouragement, Aalasi would not have information to pass on to others. Aalasi would also like to thank her daughter Joannie for helping out with interpreting throughout the project and during the sewing lessons when this project was conceived.

ᐋᓇ ᖁᔭᓐᓇᒦᖅᑐᖅ ᓃᑦ ᑯᕆᔅᑕᕗᕐᒧᑦ ᑖᓐᓇ ᐅᖅᑲᓕᒫᒐᖅ ᓴᖅᑭᒍᓐᓇᕐᓂᕿᖅᑐᓂᐅᒃ ᐅᑉᐱᕈᓯᓕᖅᑎᓚᐅᕐᒪᒍ ᐃᑲᔪᐃᓐᓇᖅᑐᓂᐅᑦᓗ ᓴᓇᔭᐅᓂᖕᒐᓂ. ᐋᓇᐅᑉ ᖁᔭᒋᑦᓚᑦᑖᕐᒥᔭᖕᒋᑦ ᖃᑕᙳᑎᖕᒋᑦ ᐱᖃᓐᓇᕆᔭᖕᒋᑦᓗ ᑲᔪᖕᒋᖅᓴᐃᑦᑎᐊᖕᒋᓐᓇᖅᐸᓚᐅᕐᒪᑕ ᐱᓇᓱᐊᕐᓂᓕᒫᖕᒐᓂ.

Anna thanks Neil Christopher for convincing her that this project was possible and for helping her make it happen. Anna would also like to thank her family and friends for the much-needed encouragement along the way.

ᕇᐱᒃ ᖁᔭᓐᓇᒦᖅᑐ ᐊᖕᒐᔪᖅᑳᖕᒋᓐᓂᓂᑦ ᐃᓄᒃᑎᑐᑦ ᐅᖅᑐᓯᕐᒥᑦ ᖃᐅᔨᒪᑎᑕᐅᒐᒥ ᐊᒻᒪᓗ ᐱᕈᖅᑐᑦ ᒥᒃᓵᓄᑦ ᐃᓕᓐᓂᐊᖅᑎᑕᐅᖅᑲᑦᑕᓚᐅᕿᒥ ᓯᕈᓯᐅᑎᑦᑐᒍ. ᖁᔭᓐᓇᒦᕐᒥᔭᖕᒋᑦ ᐸᓂᖕᒋᒃ, ᐱᖃᓐᓇᕆᔭᖕᒋᑦ, ᐊᒻᒪᓗ ᐊᖕᒋᔪᖕᒋᑦ ᑲᔪᖕᒋᖅᓴᐃᑦᑎᐊᖅᑲᑦᑕᓚᐅᖅᓂᖕᒋᑦ ᐱᓕᕆᓇᓯᑦᑎᑦᑐᒍ ᐊᔾᔨᒦᖕᒋᕈᓘᔭᖅᑐᓂᑦ.

Rebecca thanks her parents for keeping her Inuktitut strong and for teaching her about plants as a youth. She also thanks her children, friends, and sisters for supporting her through her many busy projects.

ᓴᓇᔭᐅᓂᖓ ᓴᖅᑭᑕᐅᓂᖓᓗ ᑖᒃᓯᒪ ᐅᖃᓕᒫᒐᐅᑉ ᐊᔪᙱᑎᑕᐅᓚᐅᖅᑐᖅ ᐃᓕᖅᑯᓯᓕᕆᔨᒃᑯᓐᓂᑦ ᐊᒻᒪᓗ ᑲᓇᑕᒥᑦ ᐃᓕᖅᑯᓯᖁᖅᑲᓕᕆᔨᒃᑯᓐᓂᑦ. ᐱᓕᕆᕝᕕᓕᐊᑎᑦᑐᑕᓗ ᑲᔪᙱᖅᓴᐃᖅᑳᑕᔪᓂᑦ, ᐃᓕᓴᕆᔪᒪᒻᒥᔭᕗᑦ: ᕇᑕ ᐊᖏᐊᕈᖅ; ᔪᐋᓐ ᔅᑖᓴᓐ; ᐃᐊᓚᓐ ᓯᒡᓗᖅ; ᐹᑐᕆᒃ ᓕᑐ; ᓅᓪ ᒪᒃᑐᒪᑦ; ᐅᓘᑕ ᒫᑎᐅᓯ; ᓯᐊᓕ ᕈᔅ; ᓗᐃᔅ ᕝᓚᕼᐅᕐᑎ; ᑑᓂ ᕈᒦᑐ; ᑰᑎᔅ ᕉᓚᓐ; ᐊᒻᒪᓗ ᓄᓇᕗᒻᒥᑦ ᐃᓕᓴᐃᔨᒃᓴᓄᑦ ᐃᓕᓐᓂᐊᕐᕕᒃ.

The creation and printing of this book was supported by the Department of Culture and Heritage and by Canadian Heritage. For additional support during the project, we would also like to acknowledge: Rita Akearok, Joanne Stassen, Ellen Ziegler, Patrick Little, Noel McDermott, Ooloota Matiusi, Shelley Ross, Louise Flaherty, Tony Romito, Curtis Rowland, and the Nunavut Teacher Education Program.

ᑖᓐᓇ ᐅᖃᓕᒫᒐᖅ ᑐᕌᖅᑎᑕᐅᔪᖅ ᐃᓕᑦᑐᒪᔪᓄᑦ, ᐱᒻᒪᕆᐅᒍᓯᒃᑐᓄᑦ, ᐱᕈᖅᑐᓂᒃ ᐊᑐᖅᑕᐅᔾᔪᓯᐅᔪᕙᓂᕐᓂᒃ ᑲᔪᓯᑎᑦᑎᔪᒪᔪᓄᑦ.

This book is dedicated to all those who want to learn about, value, and continue traditional plant use.

ᐋᓚᓯ ᔫᒥ
Aalasi Joamie

ᐋᓇ ᓰᒡᓗᖅ
Anna Ziegler

ᕆᐱᑲ ᓴᐃᓐᓄ
Rebecca Hainnu

ᐱᓕᕆᐊᑦ ᒥᒃᓵᓄᑦ
About This Project

ᖃᓄᕐᓕ ᖃᐅᔨᒪᑦᑎᐊᕐᓂᐊᕋᑦᑕ ᑭᓇᐅᓂᑦᑎᓐᓂᑦ, ᐋᓚᓯ ᐊᐱᕆᔪᖅ, ᓇᒥᒥᐅᑕᐅᓂᑦᑎᓐᓂᑦ ᖃᐅᔨᒪᙱᒃᑯᑦᑕ? ᐊᓈᓇᒥᓂᑦ ᐃᓕᓐᓂᐊᖅᐸᓪᓕᐊᓪᓗᓂ, ᐋᓚᓯ ᑕᑯᓐᓇᖅᑦᑕᓚᐅᖅᑐᖅ ᐃᓕᒃᑯᐊᓕᐅᖅᐸᑦᑐᓂᓗ ᐱᕈᖅᑐᓂᑦ ᓂᕈᐊᖅᓯᐊᖑᓪᓗᓂ ᐸᓐᓂᖅᑑᒥᑦ 1940ᖏᓐᓂᑦ ᐊᒻᒪᓗ ᑭᖑᓂᐊᒍᑦ ᐊᓈᓇᐅᓕᖅᑐᓂ ᓂᐊᖁᙳᒥᑦ 1960ᓂᑦ ᐅᓪᓗᒥᒧᑦ. ᐅᖃᓕᒫᒐᕐᒥᑦ ᑕᕝᕙᓂ ᓴᖅᑭᑕᐅᕗᑦ 18 ᐱᕈᖅᑐᑦ ᒥᒃᓵᓄᑦ, ᐋᓚᓯᐅᑉ ᖃᐅᔨᒪᔭᖏᑦ ᐃᖅᑲᐅᒪᔭᖏᓪᓗ ᓇᓂᔭᐅᒡᒍᔪᑦ ᐸᓐᓂᖅᑑᒥᑦ, ᓂᐊᖁᙳᖅᒥᑦ, ᓄᓇᕗᒻᒥᓗ.

How can we know who we are, Aalasi Joamie asks, *if we don't know about where we live?* Having learned from her mother, Aalasi observed and harvested plants as a little girl in Pangnirtung in the 1940s, and later as a mother in Niaqunnguuq (Apex) from the 1960s to today. In this introductory guide to traditional plant use, Aalasi shares her life's knowledge and memories of eighteen plants commonly found around Pangnirtung, Niaqunnguuq, and across Nunavut.

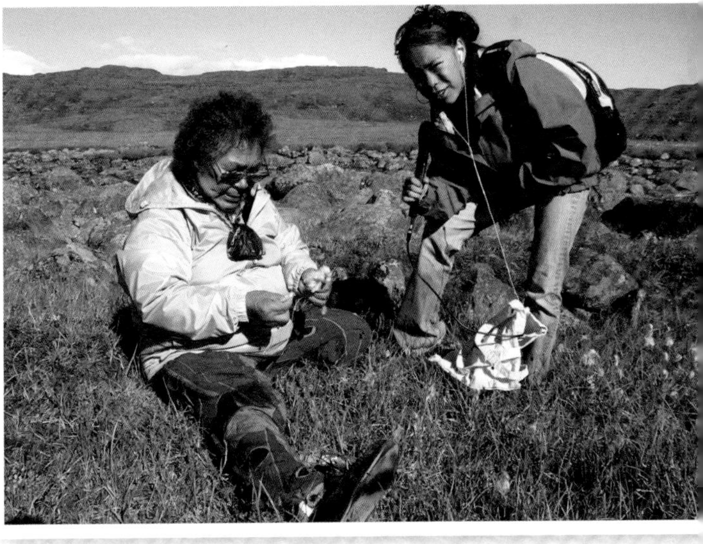

ᐋᓚᓯᒃᑯᒃ ᔫᐋᓂᒃᑯᒃ ᐃᖃᓗᐃᑦ ᑰᖓᑕ ᖃᓂᒋᔮᓂ ᖃᐅᔨᓴᖅᐸᓪᓕᐊᓪᓗᑎᒃ ᑖᒃᓱᒥᖓ ᐅᖃᓕᒫᒐᕐᒥᒃ.

Aalasi and Joannie Joamie near Iqaluit Kuunga (the Sylvia Grinnell River) during the research for this book.

ᐅᖃᓕᒫᒐᖅ ᐃᓗᓕᖅᑲᖅᐳᖅ ᐱᒋᐊᕈᑎ ᐋᓚᓯᒦᙶᖅᑐᑦ, ᓇᓗᓇᐃᒃᑯᑕᑦ ᐱᕈᖅᑐᑉ ᐊᑑᑎᖕᒋᓐᓄᑦ ᐊᑎᖕᒋᓐᓄ ᓇᓂᔭᕐᓂᕐᓂᐊᕐᒪᑕ, 18 ᐊᒡᒍᖅᓯᒪᔪᑦ ᐱᕈᖅᑐᑦ ᒥᒃᓵᓄᑦ, ᐊᒻᒪᓗ ᑎᑎᖅᓯᒪᔪᑦ ᐊᑐᒃᑲᓐᓂᖃᒃᓴᐃᑦ ᐱᕈᖅᑐᑦ ᒥᒃᓵᓅᖓᔪᑦ.

This book includes an introduction by Aalasi Joamie, a summary of the uses and names of plants for easy reference, eighteen sections on specific plants, and a list of resources for more information about the plants in this book.

ᐅᖃᓕᒫᒐᐅᑉ ᐃᓗᓕᒃᓴᖕᒋᑦ ᑲᑎᖅᓱᖅᑕᐅᓂᑯᐃᑦ ᐅᐱᖕᖓᒃᑯᑦ ᐱᓱᖃᔭᒃᑐᑎᑦ ᐃᖃᓗᐃᑦ ᑰᖓᓂ (ᓯᐅᓪᕕᐊ ᒍᕆᓂᐅᓪ) ᐊᒻᒪᓗ ᓂᐊᖁᙳᕐᒥᑦ ᐃᓚᓯᒪᓪᓗᑎᑦ ᓂᐱᓕᐅᖅᓯᒪᔫᙵᖅᑐᓂ ᐋᓚᓯᐅᑉ ᐃᓪᓗᖓᓂ. ᓯᕗᓪᓕᖅᐹᑦ ᓂᐱᓕᐅᖅᓯᒪᔪᓂᑦ ᐋᓚᓯᐅᑉ ᐅᖃᐅᓯᖕᒋᑦ ᓘᐊᑕᐅᓂᑯᑦ ᐋᓇ ᓯᒡᓗᒃᑯᓐᓂᑦ, ᐋᓚᓯᐅᓪᓗ ᐸᓂᖓ, ᔫᐊᓂ ᔫᒥ ᑐᓵᔨᐅᓪᓗᓂ, ᓂᐱᓕᐅᕈᑎᓕᕆᔨᐅᓪᓗᓂᓗ. ᑭᖑᓂᐊᒍ ᐃᓛᑉ ᐃᓄᐊᓂ ᓂᐱᓕᐅᒃᑲᓂᖅᑐᓂ. ᐊᐱᖅᓱᖅᑲᑦᑕᔪᔪᑦ ᐋᓇ ᓯᒡᓗᖅ ᐊᒻᒪᓗ ᕆᑕ ᐊᖄᐊᕈᖅ ᐃᑲᔪᖅᑎᖃᖅᑐᑎᑦ ᔪᐋᓐ ᔅᑖᓴᓐ. ᐅᐱᖕᖓᒃᑲᓐᓂᕐᒪᑦ, ᐋᓇ ᓯᒡᓗᒃᑯᑦ ᕆᐱᑲ ᕼᐊᐃᓐᓄᒃᑯᑦ ᐱᓇᓱᐊᕈᓯᓕᒫᕐᒥᑦ ᐊᐱᖅᓱᑲᓐᓂᑲᑕᒃᑐᑎᑦ ᐋᓚᓯᒥ ᐊᒻᒪ ᓂᕈᐊᖅᑐᑎᒃ ᓇᓕᐊ ᐱᕈᖅᑐᑦ ᑎᑎᖅᑕᐅᓂᐊᕐᒪᖔᑕ ᓇᓗᓇᐃᔭᐃᓪᓗᑎᒃ, ᑐᑭᓯᒋᐊᕈᑕᐅᒃᑲᓂᖅᑐᑎᓪᓗ, ᓂᐱᓕᐅᖅᑕᐅᒃᑲᓂᖅᑐᓂᓗ ᐅᖃᓪᓚᒃᑎᓪᓗᒍ ᐋᓚᓯ ᐃᓅᓯᖕᖓᑕ ᒥᒃᓵᓄᑦ. ᑎᑎᖅᑕᐅᓂᖓ ᐅᖃᓕᒫᒐᖅ ᐋᓇ ᓯᒡᓗᖅᒧᑦ ᐃᓄᒃᑎᑑᓕᖅᑎᑕᐅᓪᓗᓂ ᕆᐱᑲ ᕼᐊᐃᓐᓄᒻᒧᑦ.

The information in this book was gathered on walks around Iqaluit Kuunga (the Sylvia Grinnell River) and Niaqunnguuq, and through additional interviews in Aalasi's house. The first research interviews were conducted on walks with Aalasi by Anna Ziegler and Aalasi's daughter Joannie Joamie, who interpreted from Inuktitut to English and helped with the recording equipment. Later in the season, we conducted several interviews indoors. These interviews were conducted by Anna Ziegler and Rita Akearok, with assistance from Joanne Stassen. The following summer, Anna Ziegler and Rebecca Hainnu conducted a week of intensive interviews with Aalasi to select plants to be included in the book, gather more information, and record additional commentary by Aalasi about her life experiences. The plant sections were written by Anna Ziegler, based entirely on interview notes and transcriptions, and translated by Rebecca Hainnu.

ᐅᖃᓪᓚᒫᒐᖅ ᐃᓗᓕᓕᒃ ᐋᓚᓯᐅᑉ ᖃᐅᔨᒪᔭᖏᓐᓂᒃ, ᐃᓕᑕᕆᓂᖏᓐᓂᑦᓗ ᐊᖓᔪᖅᑳᒥᓂᑦ ᐊᓯᖏᓐᓂᓗ ᐃᓄᖕᓂᑦ ᐸᓐᓂᖅᑑᖅᒥᐅᓂᑦ ᐱᕈᖅᓴᑎᑦᓗᒍ. ᐃᓄᐃᑦ ᐊᓯᖏᑦ ᖃᐅᔨᒪᔭᖃᒃᑲᓐᓂᖅᑑᒐᓗᐊᑦ ᐊᓯᖏᓐᓂᑦ ᐊᔾᔨᒋᙱᑕᖏᓐᓂᓗ. ᐊᒻᒪᓗ ᐱᕈᖅᑐᑦ ᐊᑎᖃᐅᖅᑐᐊᓘᑦᓗᑎᑦ ᐊᔾᔩᙱᑦᑐᓂᑦ. ᐱᕈᖅᑐᑦ ᒥᒃᓴᓄᓕᒫᖂᓗᒃ ᑎᑎᕋᕋᒃᓯᒪᖏᑦᑐᒍᑦ, ᑭᓯᐊᓂᓕ ᐊᑕᐅᓯᖅᒧᑦ ᐃᓄᒻᒧᑦ ᖃᐅᔨᒪᔭᐅᕙᓂᑦ ᐊᑐᖅᑕᐅᓯᒪᕙᓂᑦ ᐸᓐᓂᖅᑑᖅᒥᑦ ᓂᐊᖁᙷᒧᑦ ᓇᓗᓇᐃᔭᐃᓇᓱᒃᓯᒪᕗᒍᑦ. ᓴᖅᑭᖁᕙᒥᓇᖅᐳᑦ ᐃᓐᓇᐃᑦ ᐊᓯᖏᑦ ᓇᑭᑐᐃᓐᓈᖅᑐᑦ ᖃᐅᔨᒪᔭᒥᓂᑦᑕᐅᖅ ᑎᑎᕋᖅᓯᒪᓗᒋᑦ ᓴᖅᑮᓗᑎᑦ ᒪᒃᑯᓐᓂᖅᓴᓄᑦ ᐊᑐᐃᓐᓇᐅᓂᖅᓴᐅᓂᐊᕐᒪᑕ ᓯᕗᓂᒃᓴᑦᑎᓐᓂᑦ.

The information in this book is a representation of Aalasi's personal knowledge, learned from her parents and other people she knew in Pangnirtung when she was growing up. Other people may know more or different things about the plants in this book and there are many other names for the plants included here. Our intention is not to present an objective body of knowledge about Arctic plants, but to record and share the subjective knowledge and experiences of one person from Pangnirtung and Niaqunnguuq. We hope that other Elders and knowledgeable community members will have opportunities to record and share their regional plant knowledge and memories so that a vibrant dialogue of Inuit traditional plant knowledge will be accessible to future generations.

ᖃᐅᔨᒪᒋᐊᕐᓂᐊᖅᐳᑎᑦ, ᐱᕈᖅᑐᑦ ᐊᒥᓱᑦ ᓴᙱᔪᒻᒪᓇᐅᒻᒪᑕ. ᐊᑐᕐᓂᐊᕐᓗᒋᑦ ᐅᔾᔨᖅᓱᑦᑎᐊᓚᐊᖃᕐᓂᐊᕋᕕᑦ! ᑕᐃᒫᑦᑎᐊᖅ ᑎᑎᕋᕋᒃᓯᒪᕙᒍ ᐅᖃᓪᓚᒫᒐᕐᒥᑦ ᑕᕝᕙᓂ ᑭᓯᐊᓂ ᐸᓯᔭᒃᓴᐅᔾᔮᙱᓚᒍᑦ ᐊᑐᑦᑎᐊᖅᑕᐅᖏᑦᓗᑎᑦ ᐊᑲᐅᕙᓐᓃᕈᑕᐅᑉᐸᑕ ᐱᕈᖅᑐᑦ. ᐃᓐᓇᑐᖃᕐᓂᑦ ᐊᐱᖅᓱᒃᑲᓐᓂᖃᑦᑕᓚᑦ ᓄᓇᒃᓯᓐᓃᑦᑐᓂᑦ ᐊᐱᖅᑯᑎᒃᓴᖃᒃᑲᓐᓂᕈᕕᑦ ᐱᕈᖅᑐᑦ ᒥᒃᓴᓄᑦ.

Please note, many plants have strong medicinal properties. Use them with care! We have done our best to provide accurate information in this book, but we do not take responsibility for any adverse effects experienced as a result of using the plants. Please talk with Elders and other knowledgeable people in the community if you have questions about local plant uses and varieties.

ᑕᑯᑎᑦᑎᒋᐊᕈᑎ ᐋᓚᓯ ᔫᒥᒦᖕᒫᖅᑐᑦ
Introduction by Aalasi Joamie

ᑖᓐᓇ ᑎᑎᕋᖅᓯᒪᔪᖅ ᐋᖅᑭᒋᐊᖅᑕᐅᓚᐅᙱᑦᑐᖅ ᐋᓚᓯᐅᑉ ᐅᖃᐅᓯᕕᓂᖏᑦ ᒪᓕᒐᓱᒃᓯᒪᔫᒐᓗᐊᑦ. ᐋᓇᒃᑯᒃ ᓃᐱᒃᑯᒃ ᐊᐱᖅᓱᓚᐅᖅᓯᒪᒻᒪᑏᒃ ᖃᓄᖅ ᐱᕈᖅᑐᑦ ᒥᒃᓵᓄᑦ ᐃᓕᓚᐅᖅᓯᒪᒻᒪᖔ, ᖃᓄᖅ ᐃᓅᓯᖓᓄᑦ ᐊᑦᑐᐃᓂᖃᖅᓯᒪᒻᒪᖔᑕ, ᖃᓄᕐᓗ ᐃᓱᒪᒻᒪᖔ ᑭᓱᑐᐃᓐᓇᐃᑦ ᐊᓯᔾᔨᖅᐸᓪᓕᐊᓂᖏᑦ ᑕᑯᓯᒪᔭᖏᑦ ᐊᑐᖅᓯᒪᔭᖏᓪᓗ ᐃᓅᓯᖓᓂᑦ. ᐊᖏᕋᖓᓂ ᔪᓚᐃ 2007ᖑᑎᓪᓗᒍ ᑎᑎᕋᖅᑕᐅᓂᑯᐃᑦ. ᓃᐱᑲᐅᓪᓗ ᓂᐱᓕᐅᖅᑕᐅᓯᒪᔪᑦ ᑎᑎᕋᖅᑐᓂᒋ ᖃᓪᓗᓈᑎᑑᓕᖅᑎᑦᑐᓂᒋᓪᓗ.

This introduction is an unedited transcript of oral commentary by Aalasi. Anna and Rebecca asked Aalasi to talk about how she learned about plants, what role plants have in her life, and how she feels about changes she has witnessed and experienced in her lifetime. It was recorded in July 2007 in her home. Rebecca transcribed the recording and translated it into English.

ᐊᓈᓇᒐ ᒪᑯᓂᖓ ᐱᕈᖅᑐᓂᑦ ᐅᓂᒃᑳᖅᑎᓪᓗᒍ, ᓂᓪᓕᐊᖅᑲᑦᑕᔭᙱᑦᑐᖓ ᓈᓚᑐᐃᓐᓇᖅᑐᒍ ᐃᒦ ᐱᐅᔫᒻᒪᑕ ᒪᑯᐊ ᐱᕈᖅᑐᑦ ᐃᒪᐃᓕᐅᖅᑲᑦᑕᓚᐅᖅᓯᒪᒻᒪᑦ. ᐱᕈᖅᑐᓂᑦ ᓄᐊᑦᑎᑎᓪᓗᒍ ᖁᕕᐊᒋᓗᐊᖅᑲᑦᑕᓚᐅᖅᓯᒪᔭᕋ ᐃᓕᒐᓱᑦᑐᖓᓗ ᐋᓐᓂᓯᐅᑎᐅᓂᕋᐃᓪᓗᓂ ᐊᒻᒪᓗ ᓂᕿᐅᓂᕋᐃᓪᓗᓂ ᐊᒻᒪ ᓂᕿᐅᖏᓐᓂᕋᐃᓪᓗᓂ ᐱᕈᖅᑐᓂ.

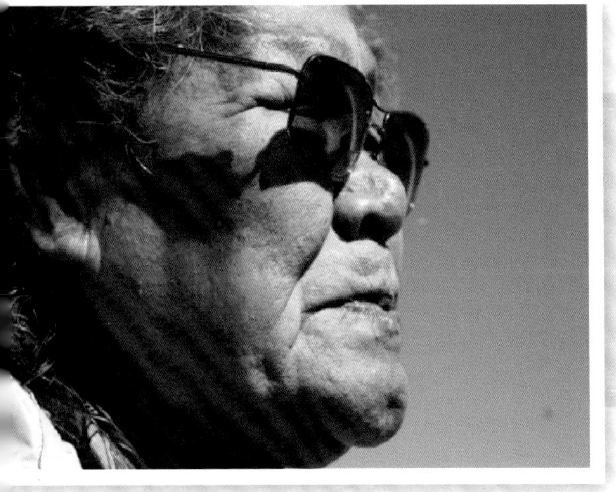

ᐋᓚᓯ ᔫᒥ ᔪᓚᐃᒥᑦ, 2006, ᐃᖅᑲᓗᐃᑦ ᑰᖓᓂᑦ (ᓯᐅᓪᕕᐊ ᒍᕆᓂᐅᓪ).

Aalasi Joamie in July 2006, near Iqaluit Kuunga (the Sylvia Grinnell River).

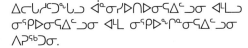

My mother taught me which plants were good. I would listen as she talked about them. I would watch my mother collecting plants. Some plants are edible and some are not. Others have medicinal uses.

ᐱᕈᖅᑐᑦ ᓂᕿᐅᓂᕋᖅᑕᖏᑦ ᓇᓗᓇᐃᖅᓯᓪᓚᕆᖅᑲᑦᑕᓚᐅᖅᓯᒪᔭᒃᑲ ᑎᑎᖅᑲᑎᒎᖏᑦᑐᖅᑕ, ᑭᓯᐊᓂ ᐃᒃᑯᐊ ᐊᕙᓃᔪᔪᖅ ᓂᖅᑮᑦ ᐃᒫ ᑕᐅᑐᒐᓯᐊᖅᑐᖓ. ᐊᒻᒪᓗ ᑎᒍᒥᐊᖏᓐᓇᖅᑲᑦᑕᔪᔪᖓ ᐅᕙᖓ ᐱᐅᕆᔭᖏᓐᓇᓂᑦ ᐱᕈᖅᑐᓂᑦ. ᑕᐃᒃᑯᐊ ᑎᒍᒥᐊᖅᑕᒃᑲ ᐱᕈᖅᑐᑦ ᐱᕈᖅᑎᒐᓯᐊᓯᑦᑕᖅᑲᒃᑲ. ᐅᑭᐅᑭᑦᑐᕈᓘᓪᓗᖓ, ᒫᓂᖅᑲᐃ ᐅᑭᐅᖅᑲᖅᑐᖓ 10, 11ᖑᔪᒃᓴᐅᓐᓂᖅᐳᖓ. ᐱᕈᖅᑎᒐᓯᐊᖅᑲᑦᑕᓚᐅᖅᓯᒪᔭᒃᑲ, ᖃᑦᑖᖅᔪᒥᓃᑦ ᖁᖑᔪᒃᓯᒪᔪᖅ ᓯᓚᒥᑦ ᓄᐊᑦᑐᕆᑦ. ᖃᖕᒑᓗᒃᑯᑦ ᖃᑦᑖᖅᔪᕕᓂᕐᒥᑦ ᑕᑯᑦᑕᓯᓐᓇᓕᖅᑲᑦᑕᖅᑐᖓ, ᖃᓪᓗᓈᖅᑲᖏᑦᑐᒦᖅᑲᑦᑕᖅᑐᑕ.

I would make mental notes about which plants were edible. I would try to remember places where they were found. I would always have plants that I liked with me. I was around ten or eleven years old when I first began to experiment with cultivating plants. I would use old tin cans for potting them. We lived in an area where there were no Qallunaat, so I only found tin cans once in a while.

ᐊᓈᓇᒐ ᕿᑦᓯᕆᑎᓪᓗᒍ ᐱᕈᖅᑎᒐᓯᐊᓯᖅᑲᑦᑕᔪᔭᒃᑲ ᐱᕈᖅᑐᑦ. ᐅᖃᐅᑎᕙᔫᒐᖓ, “ᐱᐅᒋᒍᕕᒋᑦ ᑭᓯᐊᓂ ᐱᕈᓚᖓᔪᐃᑦ, ᖁᕕᐊᒋᖏᒃᑯᕕᒋᑦ ᐱᕈᔮᖏᑦᑐᐃᑦ. ᖁᕕᐊᒋᒍᕕᒋᑦ ᑭᓯᐊᓂ”. ᑕᐃᒪ ᐱᕈᖅᐸᓪᓕᐊᖅᑲᑦᑕᕐᒪᑕ.

My mother often prepared skins while I planted flowers. She would always say to me, if you appreciate them, they will grow. If you like what you are doing, they will grow well.

ᐃᓯᒪᖅᑲᑦᑕᓯᑦᑕᕆᕗᖓ ᒫᖖᒐ ᓄᓇᑦᑎᓐᓂᑦ ᐱᐅᕆᔭᖏᓐᓂᑦ ᐅᕙᖓ ᐱᕈᖅᓯᐊᓂᑦ ᐋᖅᑭᒃᓯᐃᓗᖓ ᖃᐅᓯᖅᑐᒧᑦ ᓄᐊᑦᑐᕆᑦ. ᐃᒫ ᕿᑲᖅᓯᔭᓐᓇᑦᑎᐊᖅᑲᑦᑕᔭᖏᓐᓇᒪ, ᐱᕈᖅᓯᐊᑕᓃᓐᓇᖅᑑᔭᖅᑲᑦᑕᖅᑐᖓ ᖃᐅᔨᕙᑦᑕᐊᓯᒪᒐᒪ. ᐃᓚᖏᑦᑐ ᓂᕆᕙᑦᑐᑦ. ᐅᖅᔫᒥᐊᖅᑐᖅᐸᑦᑐᖓᓗ ᐱᕈᖅᑐᓂᑦ ᐊᓂᑯᓗᓐᓗ ᒥᓇᖅᐸᑦᑐᖓ ᐊᑯᑦᑎᖖᒍᐊᖅᑐᐊᓘᕙᑦᑐᖓᓗ ᐱᐅᓯᖏᑦᑎᐊᖅᑎᓪᓗᒍ ᐃᓚᖓᓂ ᓂᕆᕙᑦᑕᕋ, ᐃᓚᒃᑲ ᓇᖅᕈᕙᑦᑐᑦ.

Then I began to plant flowers in the moist soil. I remember I was always busy with plants. I collected them to eat and I mixed them in oil. Sometimes I would collect edible plants for my brother. Sometimes I would make *alu* (pudding) and, before it was ready, I would eat it. Not all my family members were willing to try it.

ᑕᐃᒃᑯᐊᓗ ᐱᕈᖅᓯᐊᑯᓗᐃᑦ ᒪᓕᒃᑳᑯᓗᐃᑦ, ᑕᐃᒃᑯᐊ ᓄᐊᑦᑕᖅᑲᒃᑲ. ᐊᓯᐃᑦᓛ ᐱᐅᓯᕙᑦᓚᖕᒥᓐᓇᖁᒥᑦ ᑕᐃᒫ ᐅᑕᖅᑭᑦᑎᐊᖅᓯᒪᒐᒪ ᐱᕈᖅᐸᓪᓚᐊᖕᒥᓇᖅᐸᑦᑐᑦ. ᐅᓪᓗᒥᒧᑦ ᑎᑭᑦᑐᒍ ᐱᕈᖅᑐᓖᓐᓇᖅᓯᖕᒐ. ᐃᓅᑦᑐᖕᒐ ᐱᓯᒃᓯᒪᓪᓗᖕᒐ ᐱᕈᖅᑐᐃᑦ ᐱᔾᔪᑎᒋᑦᑐᒋᑦ ᖁᔭᓇᒦᖅᑐᖕᒐ ᐊᒻᒪᓗ ᓂᕿᐅᓂᖕᒋᑦ ᐅᐱᒋᑦᑐᒋᑦ.

I would keep *malikkaat* (mountain avens) for flowers. It wasn't long before they would bloom. Throughout my life, I have been interested in plants. I have always inquired about them. When I am walking by myself, I feel thankful for all the plants. I appreciate that they are food.

ᐊᕿᐊᑦᑐᒐᓚᓷᖑᒻᒪᓇᐸᔾᔭᖕᒐ ᐱᕈᖅᑐᓂ ᓂᐸᑦᑐᖕᒐ ᖁᖑᓚᕐᓂ. ᓄᐊᐸᑦᑐᒋᑦ ᐊᒥᓱᓂᑦ ᐊᔾᔭᖅᓯᕙᔾᔭᖕᒐ. ᐃᓛ ᐱᐊᕋᖅᑲᖕᒋᒃᑲᓗᐊᕋᒪ, ᐱᐊᕋᓚᓐᓄᑦ ᑐᓂᕙᑦᑐᒋᑦ. ᑕᒪᒃᑯᐊ ᐊᔾᔪᖅᓷᔾᔭᐅᔾᔨᑎᒋᓯᒪᔭᒃᑲ ᐊᑐᕋᓱᐃᓐᓇᖅᑕᒃᑲ.

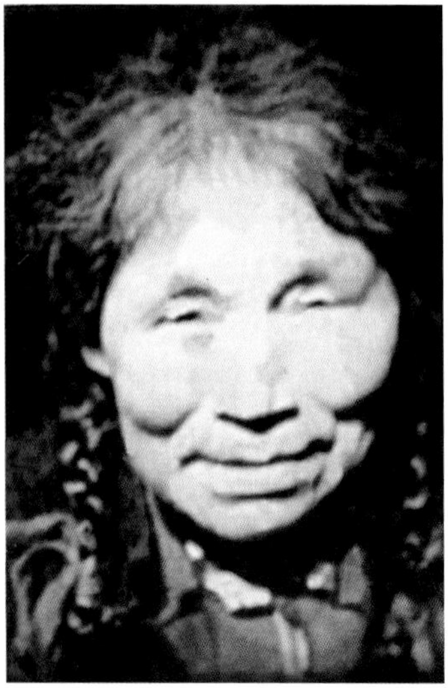

Sometimes I could get a good fill from eating plants, especially from eating *qunguliit* (mountain sorrel). I was able to collect them and carry quite a lot. Even before I had my own children, I would gather roots and give them to infants to suck on. I tried to use them as I had been taught.

ᐋᓚᓯᐅᑉ ᐊᓈᓇᖓ. ᓇᓗᔭᐅᔪᑦ ᖃᖓ ᑭᐊᓪᓗ ᐊᔾᔨᓕᐅᕐᓂᕋᒻᒪᖔᒍ. ᐊᔾᔨᙳᐊᖅ ᑐᓂᔭᐅᔪᖅ ᐋᓚᓯ ᔫᒥᒧᑦ.

Aalasi's mother. Date and photographer unknown. Photograph provided by Aalasi Joamie.

ᐅᓪᓗᒥᓕ ᐃᓐᓇᐅᓕᖅᑐᖓ ᐱᕈᖅᓯᐊᖔᓄᑦ ᖄᓯᒪᒪᒪ. ᖃᓪᓗᓈᖅᓕ ᐱᕈᖅᑐᖅᑯᑎᖏᓐᓄᑦ. ᑕᐃᒫ ᕿᓯᐊᓂᐅᔫᖅᑐᖅ ᐱᕈᖅᓯᐊᖅᑲᖅᓗᖓᐅᔫᖅᑐᖅ. ᐱᕈᖅᓯᐊᖅᑲᖏᒃᑯᒪ ᐱᔪᓐᓇᖅᑐᖅᔫᖏᑦᑐᖓ, ᐋᒡᒐᐅᓪᒥᔩᓚᓗᐊᖅ. ᐊᑦᓯᐊᓗᒃ ᐱᐅᒋᔭᒃᑲ, ᐊᑦᓯᐊᓗᒃ ᐅᕙᓐᓅᖓᔭᐃᑦ. ᑕᕝᕙ ᓱᕈᓯᐅᓪᓗᖓ ᓂᕕᐊᖅᓯᐊᖑᓪᓗᖓ, ᐅᕕᒃᑲᐅᓪᓗᖓ ᐊᒻᒪ ᐅᕕᒃᑲᕈᖅᐸᓪᓕᐊᓪᓗᖓ, ᐊᒫᖅᑲᑦᑕᓕᖅᑐᖓᓗ ᕿᑐᖖᒐᖅᑲᓕᖅᑐᖓ ᐱᕈᖅᑐᓂᑦ ᐱᕕᔾᔭᐊᖅᑲᖅᓯᒪᒪᒪ. ᑕᐃᒪ ᕿᑐᖖᒐᒃᑲ ᑕᓯᐅᖅᑐᕆᑦ ᐅᖅᑲᓚᒪᕕᒋᖅᑲᑦᑕᖅᓯᒪᔭᒃᑲ ᐱᕈᖅᑐᐃᑦ ᐱᐅᔩᓪᒪᖔᑕ ᐊᒻᒪᓗ ᐱᐅᖏᑦᑑᓪᒪᖔᑕ. ᑕᐃᒪᐃᒃᑑᖅᑲᑦᑕᖅᓯᒪᔭᖓ. ᐋᓐᓂᐊᓯᐅᑎᐅᔪᓐᓇᖅᓂᖏᑦ ᖃᐅᔨᒪᔭᒃᑲ, ᐱᐅᔪᐃᑦ ᖃᐅᔨᒪᔭᒃᑲ, ᐊᒻᒪᓗ ᐋᓐᓂᖅᓇᖅᓂᖏᑦ ᖃᐅᔨᒪᔭᒃᑲ. ᑕᒻᒪᖅᑐᕕᓂᐅᒍᒪ ᐱᓯᑦᓗᖓ ᐅᔭᖁᐃᑦ, ᐱᕈᖅᑐᐃᑦᓗ, ᑕᒻᒪᓈᒃᑯᑎᒋᓗᒋᑦ ᐊᑖᑕᒪ ᐊᔪᕆᖅᓲᔾᔨᔾᔪᑎᒋᓪᓗᓂᒋᑦ, ᑕᐃᒪᐃᒐᓯᐊᖅᑲᑦᑕᖅᓯᒪᓪᒥᔭᖓ ᑕᖅᕆᓯᒪᔭᒍᑦ ᑕᒻᒪᕋᔭᖅᒪᖔᖅᒪ ᐃᓐᓅᕈᐃᑦ, ᐊᓄᕆ ᐊᒻᒪ ᐃᕕᒃᓯᒐᐃᑦ ᐊᑐᖅᑐᒥᑦ.

As an Elder, I have turned to the plants of the Qallunaat as well. It is as if I am unable to live without plants. I really like plants. They have been a part of my childhood, my adolescence, and my motherhood. I have taken my toddlers out on walks with me. I have tried to pass on my knowledge of plants to my children. I know which plants are edible, which are harmful, and which have medicinal uses. My father also taught me how to use plants as indicators, as a compass is used. By using rocks, and the positions of plants, wind, and hills, you can find your way back. I have learned the use of these indicators through trial and error.

ᐃᔨᒧᑦ ᐊᑐᖅᑐᑦ ᐃᔨᓯᐅᑏᑦ ᐊᑐᕿᓱᖅᑲᑦᑕᖅᓯᒪᔭᒃᑲ. ᓲᕈᓗᓗᐊᖅᑐᖓᓗ ᒪᓃᑦ ᓂᕆᖅᑲᑦᑕᖅᓯᒪᔭᒃᑲ ᐋᖅᑭᒍᑎᒋᓇᓱᒃᑐᒥᑦ. ᓂᖅᓇᐃᓗ ᖃᐅᔨᒪᓪᒥᔭᒃᑲ ᐋᓐᓂᐊᓯᐅᑎᐅᔪᓐᓇᖅᑐᖅ. ᐊᓈᓇᒐ ᐅᕙᓐᓂᑦ ᖃᐅᔨᑎᑦᑎᖅᑲᑦᑕᖅᓯᒪᖏᑉᐸ ᖃᐅᔨᒪᒐᔭᙱᑕᒃ. ᐅᕙᓐᓂᑦ ᐃᓕᓐᓂᐊᖅᑎᑦᑏᓐᓇᖅᑲᑦᑕᔪᓪᒪ ᖃᐅᔨᒪᓚᖅᑭᔭᒃ ᐅᓂᒃᑳᖏᓇᖅᑲᑦᑕᔪᓪᒪ ᐱᓯᑐᓄᒃ. ᒪᕐᕈᐃᓐᓇᐅᖏᒃᑲᓗᐊᖅᑐᓄ ᐃᓛᓐᓂᓗ ᒪᕐᕈᐃᓐᓇᐅᓪᓗᓄ ᐱᓯᑉᐸᓚᐅᖅᑐᒍᑦ, ᐅᔾᔨᖅᓱᐃᓐᓇᑦᑎᐊᖁᓯᐊᖅᐸᑦᑐᖓ.

I have used *ijisiuti* (river algae) to relieve a sore eye. I have used *maniq* (lamp moss) to relieve heartburn. I know that *nirnait* (snow lichen) has medicinal uses. My mother taught me these things. If she had not shown me these things, I would not know them. Sometimes we would walk by ourselves and other times we had company, but I always paid attention.

ᐊᓈᓇᒪ ᐊᒥᓱᓂᑦ ᐊᔪᕆᖅᓲᑎᕙᔪᒻᒪᖓ. ᓲᕐᓗ, ᐃᖃᓗᐃᑦ ᒎᒥᑦ ᓇᒧᙵᓲᖑᒻᒪᙶᑕ ᐊᒻᒪᓗ ᓱᓲᖑᒻᒪᙶᑕ. ᖃᓄᓕᒫᑦᑎᐊᖅ ᐊᓈᓇᒪ ᐊᔪᕆᖅᓲᑎᓯᒪᒑᖓ.

My mother taught me about many things. From her, I learned where the char fry go when they grow up and what they do. My mother taught me about everything.

ᐱᕈᖅᓴᓯᒪᒐᒪ ᐸᓐᓂᖅᑑᒥ. ᐅᑭᐅᑭᑦᑐᕈᓘᑦᑐᖓ ᐸᓐᓂᖅᑑᒨᖅᑐᑕ. ᑭᓯᐊᓂᓕ ᕿᑐᙵᖃᓕᖅᑐᖓ ᐱᖓᓱᓂᑦ ᒪᐅᙵᓕᓚᐅᖅᓯᒪᔪᒍ (ᓂᐊᖁᙴᒧᑦ) ᐅᑭᐊᒃᓵᕌᓗᒃᑯᑦ, ᐃᒃᑮᕐᓇᖅᓯᔪᐊᓘᑎᑦᑐᒍ. ᑭᓯᐊᓂ ᐊᔾᔨᒋᑕᓚᐅᖅᓯᒪᙱᑦᑕᖅ ᒪᐅᙵᒐᑦᑕ.

We moved to Pangnirtung when I was very young. It was not until I had three children that we moved here [to Niaqunnguuq (Apex)]. We moved here in the fall, when the weather was becoming very cold. It was very different here.

ᑐᙵᓱᐃᓐᓇᖅᑐᐊᓘᑦᑐᖓ ᐃᓕᕋᓱᙱᑦᑎᐊᖅᑐᖓ ᐊᓯᔾᔨᖅᑐᐊᓘᑳᑦᓚᒃᑐᖓ, ᖁᕕᐊᓇᖅᑐᐃᓐᓇᐅᔮᖅᑐᑎᑦ. ᑭᓯᐊᓂᓗ ᐃᓚᒃᑲ ᕿᒪᒍᒪᖏᒃᑲᓗᐊᖅᑐᒋᑦ. ᓱᓇᐅᕝᕙ ᑕᑯᒃᑲᓐᓂᔾᔮᒍᓐᓃᖅᑐᒋᑦ ᐊᓈᓇᒃᑯᒃᑲ. ᐊᓯᔾᔨᑳᑦᓚᑦᑐᐊᓘᔭᓚᐅᖅᓯᒪᔪᖅ. ᕿᐊᖃᑦᑕᓚᐅᖅᓯᒪᒐᒪ ᐃᓚᓐᓅᕈᒪᑦᓗᖓ, ᑭᓯᐊᓂ ᑐᙵᓱᓚᖓᔪᐊᓘᑦᓗᑕ.

People were kind and willing to help us out through gifts. I was no longer afraid. I then had confidence. Everything was exciting. However, there were times when I cried, longing for my family. I never saw my mother again.

ᑕᒪᓐᓇᓗ ᐃᓕᓯᒪᓇᒍ ᓄᓇ, ᐃᓄᖏᑦᓗ ᐃᓕᓯᒪᓇᒋᑦ. ᓱᓇᐅᕝᕙ ᐊᖏᕐᕋᕈᒪᔾᔮᒍᓐᓃᖅᑐᖓ, ᑕᑉᐸᐅᙵᕈᒪᔾᔮᖏᑦᑐᖓ. ᑕᐃᒪ ᐊᒃᓱᕈᕐᓇᖅᑐᒃᑰᖅᐸᓕᓚᐅᖅᓯᒪᔪᖓ ᐃᓐᓇᕈᖅᐸᑦᓕᐊᓕᖅᑐᖓ ᕿᑐᙵᒃᑲᓗ ᐊᒥᓱᕈᖅᐸᑦᓕᐊᓕᖅᑐᑎᒃ. ᐃᓚᒃᑲᓗ ᓇᔪᖅᑎᒋᓇᒋᑦ. ᑭᓯᐊᓂ ᐊᔪᕐᓇᖅᑐᒃᑰᕋᓗᐊᕋᑦᑕ ᐱᔪᓐᓇᖅᑕᒃᑰᖏᓐᓇᖅᑎᑕᐅᖃᑦᑕᓚᐅᖅᓯᒪᔪᒍ.

We were very well received here. I was in an unfamiliar land with unfamiliar people. But in the end, I would never long to go back up there [to Pangnirtung]. I was never homesick again. When I got older and had more children, I went through hardships. I had to persevere without the support of my extended family because I did not live close to them. Fortunately, we were able to endure those hardships.

ᑖᒃᑯᐊ ᕿᑐᕐᖓᒃᑲ ᐱᕈᖅᐸᓪᓕᐊᓕᖅᑎᓪᓗᒋᑦ ᐅᖃᐅᑎᖃᑦᑕᓚᐅᖅᓯᒪᔭᒃᑲ ᐱᕈᖅᑐᐃᑦ ᖃᓄᖅ ᐊᑐᖅᑕᐅᓲᖑᒻᒪᖔᑕ ᐊᒻᒪᓗ ᐊᐅᓪᓚᖅᓯᒪᓗᑎᑦ ᓂᕿᒃᓴᐃᒍᓐᓂᖓᓗᐊᕈᑎᑦ ᐱᕈᖅᑐᓂᑦ ᓂᕿᒃᓴᖃᕈᓐᓇᖏᓱᐊᖅᑯᓪᓗᒋᑦ.

As my children were growing up, I taught them about plants. During camping trips, I showed them which plants were edible and which ones were not. I wanted them to know that if they ever got stranded on the land, they could draw upon many resources available to them.

ᑕᐃᒪ ᒫᓐᓇᐅᓕᖅᑐᖅ ᐅᕙᒃᑲᐃᑦ ᖃᐅᔨᒪᓕᕐᒋᑦᑎᐊᓕᖅᒪᑕ, ᐅᕙᒃᑲᐅᕐᒋᑦᑑᒐᓗᐊᑦ ᑕᒪᓐᓇ ᓂᕿᒃᓴᖅᑕᖃᒻᒪᖔᑦ ᓄᓇᒥᑦ ᐱᕈᖅᑐᓂᑦ. ᐱᑕᓕᐊᓘᑎᓪᓗᒍ, ᐅᔾᔨᕆᑦᑎᐊᖑᓯᐊᖅᓗᒋᑦ ᑲᒪᒋᓗᒋᑦ ᑕᒪᓐᓇ ᓂᕆᔭᒃᓴᖅᑕᓕᐊᓗ ᓄᓇᒥ. ᐃᒫ ᓂᕆᔭᒃᓴᖅᑕᓕᐊᓘᔭᕐᒋᑦᑑᒐᓗᐊᖅ ᓂᕿᑦᓴᕆᐊᓗᓐᓂᑦ. ᑭᓯᐊᓂ ᓂᕆᔭᒃᓴᖅᑕᖃᒻᒪᑦ ᐃᒫ ᐆᑦᑐᒋᑦ ᐊᒻᒪ ᓂᕆᑐᐃᓐᓇᖏᓗᐊᖅᑐᒋᑦ. ᐱᐅᓪᓗᓂᓗ ᓄᓇ ᐊᒻᒪ ᕿᐅᓪᓗᓂ ᐅᖅᑰᔾᔭᑎᒃᓴᖅᑕᓕ. ᐊᔭᕆᖅᓲᑎᒋᐊᒃᑲᓐᓂᖅᐸᒃᑲ ᐅᕙᒃᑲᐃᑦ. ᑕᒻᒪᖅᓯᒪᓕᖅᓂᕈᒃᓯᑦ ᓇᒦᓪᓗᓯ, ᕿᔪᒃᑕᖅᓯᒪᓗᓯ ᓄᐊᑦᑎᓯᒪᓗᓯ. ᐊᒻᒪᓗ ᐃᓐᓈᕈᔾᔫᒃ ᓴᓂᐊᓂ ᐅᖅᑯᐊᓕᓂᖅᒥᑦ ᕿᓂᖅᓗᓯ ᐊᑐᖅᑐᐃᑦ. ᐅᕙᒃᑲᐅᔪᓯ ᐅᖃᐅᑎᒋᐊᖅᐸᒃᓯ. ᐊᓄᓕᒧᑦ ᓲᖕᖓᕐᒋᓪᓗᒍ ᐅᖅᑯᐊᒧᑦ ᓲᖕᖓᖕᖔᖅᓗᑎ ᐊᒡᒍᖅᑕᐃᓕᓗᓯ.

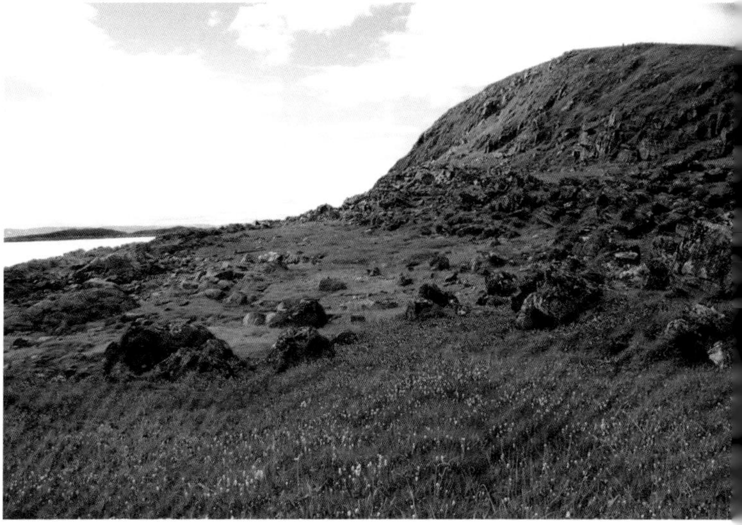

ᒥᕐᒎᐃᖅᓯᖅᕕᒻᒥᑦ ᓂᐊᖁᙴᒥᑦ (ᐊᐃᐸᒃᔅ), ᑖᒪᓂᑦ ᐋᓚᓯ ᐃᓕᒃᑯᐊᓕᐅᓕᖅᑐᖅ ᑕᐃᒪᙵ ᓅᓚᐅᖅᓯᒪᒐᒥᑦ ᐸᓐᓂᖅᑑᒥᑦ 1960ᖏᓐᓂᑦ.

Coastal park in Niaqunnguuq (Apex), where Aalasi has harvested plants since she moved from Pangnirtung in the 1960s.

Now, young and old alike seem to be ignorant about tundra vegetation. They do not seem to realize that there is a lot of food out there. I know it must look like there is not much food, but there is. We must notice the plants and we must look after them well. There are foods out there that we can cook or eat after we pick them. Plants are healthy for us. I am talking to the younger generation now. Plants can be used as survival tools. For example, if you get lost during a hike, you can pick *qijuktaat* (white heather) for a mattress. Go behind a rock or ditch facing away from the wind and use the qijuktaat for warmth.

ᐊᒻᒪ ᑰᒻᒥᑦ ᐃᑳᕈᓐᓇᐃᓕᐅᖅᑲᖅᑕᐃᓕᓗᓯ. ᓯᑕᓗᓲᕌᓗᒻᒪᑦ ᓯᑕᓗᑦᑐᖅᐹᓘᑕᐅᖅᑎᓐᓇᒍ ᐃᑳᓇᐊᖅᑲᑦᑕᕐᓗᓯ. ᓯᑕᓗᕐᑖᖅᑎᑦᓗᒍ ᐃᑳᕈᓐᓇᐃᓕᓲᕌᓘᒐᑦᑕ. ᐅᑯᐊᑦᑕᐅᖅ ᖃᐅᔨᓴᑦᑎᐊᕐᑲᑦᑕᕐᓗᒋᑦ ᑰᒃ, ᐊᒻᒪ ᑎᓂᓐᓂᖅ ᐊᒻᒪ ᐱᑐᕐᓂᐊᓗᒃ. ᑕᒪᒃᑯᐊ ᖃᐅᔨᓴᕆᐊᕐᑲᖅᑕᐃᓐᓇᕆᓚᑦᑎᒍ. ᐊᑏᓗ ᐱᕈᖅᑐᓂ ᖃᐅᔨᔪᒪᒍᑦᓯ ᐊᐱᖅᓱᕈᓐᓇᖅᑲᑦᑕᕋᔭᖅᑐᓯ ᐅᕙᓐᓂᑦᓘᓐᓃᑦ ᑕᒪᒃᑯᐊ ᖃᐅᔨᒪᒐᒃᑭᑦ ᐱᕈᖅᑐᐃᑦ ᐊᒻᒪᓗ ᑭᓱᐃᓐᓇᐃᑦ.

I would also like people to know that they should not be scared to cross rivers. They should try to cross rivers before the rain. Rivers can become very deep after it rains, so people should try to cross them as soon as they can. I think people should become more aware of the behaviour of tides, full moons, and rivers. If you want to learn more about plants and other things, ask people who know about them, like I do. I know about other things, too.

ᐃᓐᓇᐅᓕᖅᐸᑦᑕᐊᓕᖅᑎᑦᓗᖕᒐᓕ ᐊᑐᖅᓯᒪᕗᖕᒐ ᑕᒪᒃᑯᓂᖕᒐ. ᐱᕈᖅᐸᑦᑕᐊᓂᐊᖅᑐᓯ ᖃᐅᔨᓴᕐᑕᐊᕆᐊᖅᓂᐊᖅᑐᓯ ᖃᓄᕈᓘᔭ ᐱᕈᖅᑐᐃᑦ ᖃᓄᐃᑦᑑᒻᒪᖔᑕ ᐊᒻᒪᓗ ᑕᒻᒪᖅᓯᒪᓕᖅᑎᑦᓗᑕ ᓄᓇᒥᑦ ᓇᒧᑦ ᓵᖖᒐᒋᐊᖅᒪᖔᑦᑕ, ᓇᐅᒃᑯᑦᓗ ᒪᔪᓇᐊᖅᒪᖔᑦᑕ, ᐊᖅᑲᓇᐊᖅᒪᖔᑕᓗ. ᐅᓕᔾᔪᐅᓃᑦ, ᐅᓕᓐᓂᖅ ᖃᐅᔨᓴᑦᑎᐊᕐᓗᒋᑦ ᐊᒻᒪᓗ ᐱᕈᖅᑐᓂᑦ ᐱᕈᖅᑎᐊᓲᖕᒍᓂᖕᒥ ᐊᒻᒪ ᐊᓐᓂᐊᓯᐅᑎᐅᓂᖕᒋᓐᓂᑦ. ᑕᐃᓖᒐᓚᒃ.

Growing up, I was immersed in the knowledge of plants. You must take the time to learn about them. You should know which plant does what. They can help you find your way if you are lost on the tundra. They are indicators of direction. But, also, you can use them to identify areas where it is safe to climb up or down. You must also learn about the high tide, such as when and where it occurs. You should learn about the different uses of plants, which ones are edible and which ones are used for medicine. These are the sorts of things you should learn.

ᒪᑯᓂᖓ ᐊᓯᔾᔨᖅᐸᓪᓕᐊᓕᖅᑐᓂᑦ ᐅᔾᔨᕈᓱᓗᐊᙳᐊᖅᓯᒪᔪᖓ ᒪᐅᙵᔪᒐᑦᑕᓂᑦ ᓂᐊᖁᙴᒧᑦ. ᒪᐅᙵᔪᒐᑦᑕ ᖃᕐᒪᖃᔪᒐᑦᑕ ᐅᐱᓐᓇᕋᓂ ᐃᓪᓗᓕᓪᓚᑎᐊᓗᑦᑕᖃᔪᖏᒻᒪᓪᓕ. ᑕᐃᑲᓂ ᖃᕐᒦᑦᑐᑕ ᐃᓪᓗᑖᓛᕐᓂᐊᕐᓂᕋᑦᑕ ᐃᓱᒪᓚᐅᖅᓯᒪᔪᖓ ᓱᕐᕋᒍᒪᓇᖓ ᖃᕐᒦᓐᓂᕋ ᐱᐅᔪᐊᓘᒻᒪᑦ. ᑭᓯᐊᓂ ᒐᕙᒪᒃᑯᑦ ᑕᐃᒫ ᐱᖁᔨᓚᐅᖅᓯᒪᒻᒪᑕ ᐃᓪᓗᑖᕐᓗᑕ ᑭᓯᐊᓂ. ᖁᕕᐊᓇᓚᐅᖅᓯᒪᖏᑦᑐᕐᓕ ᐃᓪᓗᑖᕐᓂᐊᓕᕋᑦᑕ, ᖃᐅᔨᒪᓇᕐᒐ ᐃᓪᓗᑦ ᖃᓄᖅ ᐱᔭᐅᓲᖑᒻᒪᖖᒑᑕ.

I began to see many changes when we moved here [to Niaqunnguuq]. We were still living in a *qarmaq* (sod house) when we moved here. The first real change I experienced was moving into a house. I wanted to remain in my qarmaq, but the government forced us to move into a house. I was not happy about this. I had no idea how to live in a house.

ᑭᓯᐊᓂ ᖁᕕᐊᓇᖏᑦᑐᒧᑦ ᑎᑭᒃᑲᓗᐊᕋᑦᑕ ᕿᓄᐃᓵᕋᓯᐊᖅᑕᖁᔭᐅᓯᒪᒐᑦᑕ ᐊᖓᔪᖅᑳᑦᑎᓐᓄᑦ ᑕᒪᒃᑯᐊ ᑭᓱᑐᐃᓐᓇᐃᑦ ᐅᖁᑎᓐᓅᒐᓗᐊᖅᐸᑕ. ᑕᐃᒪᐃᒐᓱᐊᑐᐃᓐᓇᓚᐅᖅᓯᒪᔪᖓᓕ. ᑐᐊᕕᓗᐊᕋᓱᐊᖅᑕᖁᔨᖏᑦᑐᖓ ᐃᓱᒪᓂᑦ ᑎᑭᑕᐅᒐᓗᐊᕈᔾᔨ ᐊᔾᔨᒌᖏᑦᑐᓄᑦ. ᐊᔾᔨᐅᒍᓐᓃᕋᓗᐊᖅᐸᑦ ᐊᑐᖅᑕᓯᑦ, ᐊᑐᖅᑕᐅᔪᓄᑦ ᐊᓯᑦᑎᓐᓄᑦ. ᐊᔾᔨᒋᓕᓴᕚ ᑕᕝᕙ ᐊᑐᖅᑕᐅᖁᔭᐅᔪᖅ, ᐃᒪᐃᓕᐅᖅᑐᖃᕋᓗᐊᖅᑎᑦᓗᒍ ᑭᓯᐊᓂ ᐅᐃᒪᔾᔮᓴᐊᖃᖏᑦᑐᓯ. ᐅᖃᐅᔾᔭᐅᖃᑦᑕᔪᒐᑦᑕᓕ ᐊᖓᔪᖅᑳᑦᑎᓐᓄᑦ ᐱᓛᖅᑐᑦ ᖃᓄᐃᑦᑐᖃᓛᖅᑐᓂ ᐅᖃᖅᐸᔪᒻᒪᑕ. ᑕᐃᒪᐃᑐᐃᓐᓇᒧᑦᓕ ᑲᐹᖅᓯᒪᓪᓗᐊᖃᑦᑕᔪᒐᑦᑕ ᐊᓯᒋᓕᕋᓗᐊᖅᑎᑦᓗᒍ ᐃᓅᓯᖅ. ᐃᓪᓗᑖᖅᑐᑕᓗ, ᐃᑯᒪᖃᓕᖅᑐᑕ ᐊᒻᒪᓗ ᐅᐊᓵᕐᕕᖃᓕᖅᑐᑕ ᐅᖃᓚᐅᑎᑖᖅᐸᓪᓕᐊᓪᓗᑕᓗ. ᑕᒪᒃᑯᐊ ᑭᓯᐊᓂ ᖁᕕᐊᓇᓚᐅᕋᓗᐊᖅᑐᑎᑦ ᖁᕕᐊᓇᕈᓐᓃᖅᐸᓪᓕᐊᓕᓚᐅᖅᓯᒪᒻᒥᔪᖅ ᐊᑭᑦᑐᖅᐸᓪᓕᐊᓂᐊᓗᖏᑦ ᐱᔾᔪᑎᒋᓪᓗᒋᑦ.

I always tried to be prudent in how I encountered the many changes that followed that one. Our parents taught us not to rush into making decisions. They told us to take our time and to have clear minds. This is how I kept my composure through the many changes that occurred. We were warned about the changes to come, and I think this is why I was never shocked by them. Along with the house, soon came washing machines, electricity, and the telephone. Although these changes were fascinating at first, they also came with financial burdens.

ᐅᑦᑐᒥᑦ ᐊᓯᔾᔨᖅᐸᓪᓚᐊᖏᓐᓇᖅᑐᑦ. ᑕᐃᒪᐃᒃᑲᓗᐊᖅᑎᓪᓗᒍ ᒪᑭᑕᒐᓱᐊᖏᓐᓇᖅᓯᒪᔪᒍᑦ. ᐅᑦᑐᒥ ᓵᓚᐅᒐᓱᐊᖅᑲᑕᖏᑦᑐᒍ ᐱᓕᑦᑕᐊᔫᒐᓗᐊᓄᑦ, ᖃᑦᑐᓈᓂᖖᒑᖅᑑᒐᓗᐊᓂ ᐅᓕᒍ ᐃᓅᓯᓇᑦᑕᐅᑎᒥᖖᒋᑕᖏᓐᓂᑦ. ᑭᓯᐊᓂ ᑕᒪᒃᑯᓄᖓ ᐅᐸᑐᐃᔭᐅᓇᐊᖅᑲᖏᑦᑐᓯ, ᓄᑲᖅᑏ ᐅᓕᓐᓂᑦ ᐅᖃᐅᑎᒋᐊᖅᐸᔅᓯ ᑕᐃᒪᐃᑦᑐᓄ ᑎᑭᑕᐅᕖᖁᓗᐊᕈᒃᓯᑦ ᐅᐸᓘᖅᑲᑦᑕᐃᓚᒋᔅᓯ ᐃᓅᓯᑦᓯᓐᓂᑦ, ᑕᐃᒪᐃᖅᑲᑦᑕᖅᑯᔭᐅᓯᒪᓚᑦᑕ.

I am telling the younger people now that they must be prepared for change. Do not get lost in the rapid changes in our lives. Many things come from the Qallunaat that are not in our traditional customs. We must be prepared for these changes. Be prepared as we have been taught to be prepared.

ᐋᓚᓯ ᔫᒥ
ᓂᐊᖁᙱᖅ, ᓄᓇᕗᑦ, 2007

Aalasi Joamie
Niaqunnguuq (Apex), Nunavut, 2007

ᓇᓗᓇᐃᒃᑯᑕᑦ ᐱᕈᖅᑐᑦ ᐊᑑᑎᖏᓐᓄᑦ ᐊᑎᖏᓐᓄᓗ
Summary of Plant Uses and Names

ᐃᓄᒃᑎᑐᑦ **Inuktitut**	ᖃᓪᓗᓈᑎᑐᑦ **English**	ᐊᑑᑎᖏᑦ **Uses**	ᓈᓴᐅᑎᖓ **Page**
ᐊᓚᒃᓴᐅᔭᐃᑦ Alaksaujait	Net-vein willow	ᑏᖔᒍᐊᖅ, ᓂᕿ, ᐃᑭᐊᖅᑎᒃᓴᖅ, ᒪᓂᖅ Tea, food, insulation, wick	43
ᐃᔾᓯᐅᑎ Ijisiuti	River algae	ᐊᑲᐅᓯᓴᐅᑎᑦ Medicine	105
ᑲᓪᓚᐃᑦ ᑲᓪᓚᖅᑯᑎᓪᓗ Kallait kallaqutillu	Bearberry	ᓂᕿᑦ, ᑏᖔᒍᐊᑦ Food, tea	72
ᑭᒍᑕᖏᕐᓇᐃᑦ ᓇᖅᑯᑎᓪᓗ Kigutangirnait naqutillu	Blueberry	ᓂᕿᑦ Food	75
ᒪᓕᒃᑳᑦ Malikkaat	Mountain avens	ᓯᑕᒧᑦ, ᓄᓇᐅᑉᓗ ᑭᓱᑯᑦᑎᐊᓃᓂᖓᓂ ᖃᐅᔨᒪᔾᔪᑎᑦ Navigation, weather, medicine	93
ᒪᓂᖅ Maniq	Lamp moss	ᒪᓂᖅ, ᐊᑲᐅᓯᓴᐅᑎᑦ Wick, medicine	29
ᓂᕐᓇᐃᑦ Nirnait	Snow lichen	ᐊᑲᐅᓯᓴᐅᑎᑦ Medicine	109
ᐸᐅᓐᓇᐃᑦ Paunnait	Dwarf fireweed	ᓂᕿᑦ, ᑏᖔᒍᐊᑦ, ᐊᑲᐅᓯᓴᐅᑎᑦ Tea, food, medicine	47

ᐃᓄᒃᑎᑐᑦ **Inuktitut**	ᖃᓪᓗᓈᑎᑐᑦ **English**	ᐊᑑᑎᖏᑦ **Uses**	ᓈᓯᐅᑎᖓ **Page**
ᐸᐅᕐᖓᐃᑦ ᐸᐅᕐᖓᖁᑎᓪᓗ Paurngait paurngaqutillu	Crowberry	ᓂᕿᑦ Food	68
ᐳᐊᓗᙳᐊᑦ Pualunnguat	Arctic cotton	ᒪᓂᖅ, ᓴᓗᒻᒪᖅᓴᐅᑎᑦ, ᐃᑭᐊᖅᑎᒃᓴᑦ Wick, cleaner, insulation	23
ᐳᔪᐊᓗᒃ Pujualuk	Dried mushroom	ᐊᑲᐅᓯᓴᐅᑎᑦ Medicine	113
ᕿᔪᒃᑖᖅᐸᐃᑦ Qijuktaaqpait	Labrador tea	ᐊᑲᐅᓯᓴᐅᑎᑦ Medicine	81
ᖁᐊᕋᐃᑦ Quarait	Snow-bed willow	ᓂᕿᑦ Food	39
ᖁᖑᓖᑦ Qunguliit	Mountain sorrel	ᓂᕿᑦ, ᐊᑲᐅᓯᓴᐅᑎᑦ Food, medicine	55
ᓴᐸᖓᕋᓛᙳᐊᑦ ᑐᖅᑕᐃᓪᓗ Sapangaralaannguat tuqtaillu	Alpine bistort	ᓂᕿᑦ Food	61
ᓯᐅᕋᐅᑉ ᐅᖃᐅᔭᖏᑦ Siuraup uqaujangit	Seaside bluebells	ᓂᕿᑦ, ᐊᑲᐅᓯᓴᐅᑎᑦ Food, medicine	87

ᐃᓄᒃᑎᑐᑦ **Inuktitut**	ᖃᑦᓗᓈᑎᑐᑦ **English**	ᐊᑑᑎᖏᑦ **Uses**	ᓈᓴᐅᑎᖓ **Page**
ᐅᖅᐱ ᓱᐳᑎᓪᓗ Uqpi suputillu	Arctic willow	ᑏᖖᒍᐊᑦ, ᓂᕿᑦ, ᐊᑲᐅᓯᔭᐅᑎᑦ, ᐃᑭᐊᖅᑎᒃᓴᑦ, ᒪᓂᖅ Tea, food, medicine, insulation, wick	33
ᐅᕐᔪ Urju	Peat moss	ᖁᑦᑕᕐᕕᑦ, ᐃᑭᐊᖅᑎᒃᓴᑦ, ᒪᓂᖅ Diapers, insulation, wick	99

ᐱᐅᖅᑐᑦ
Plants

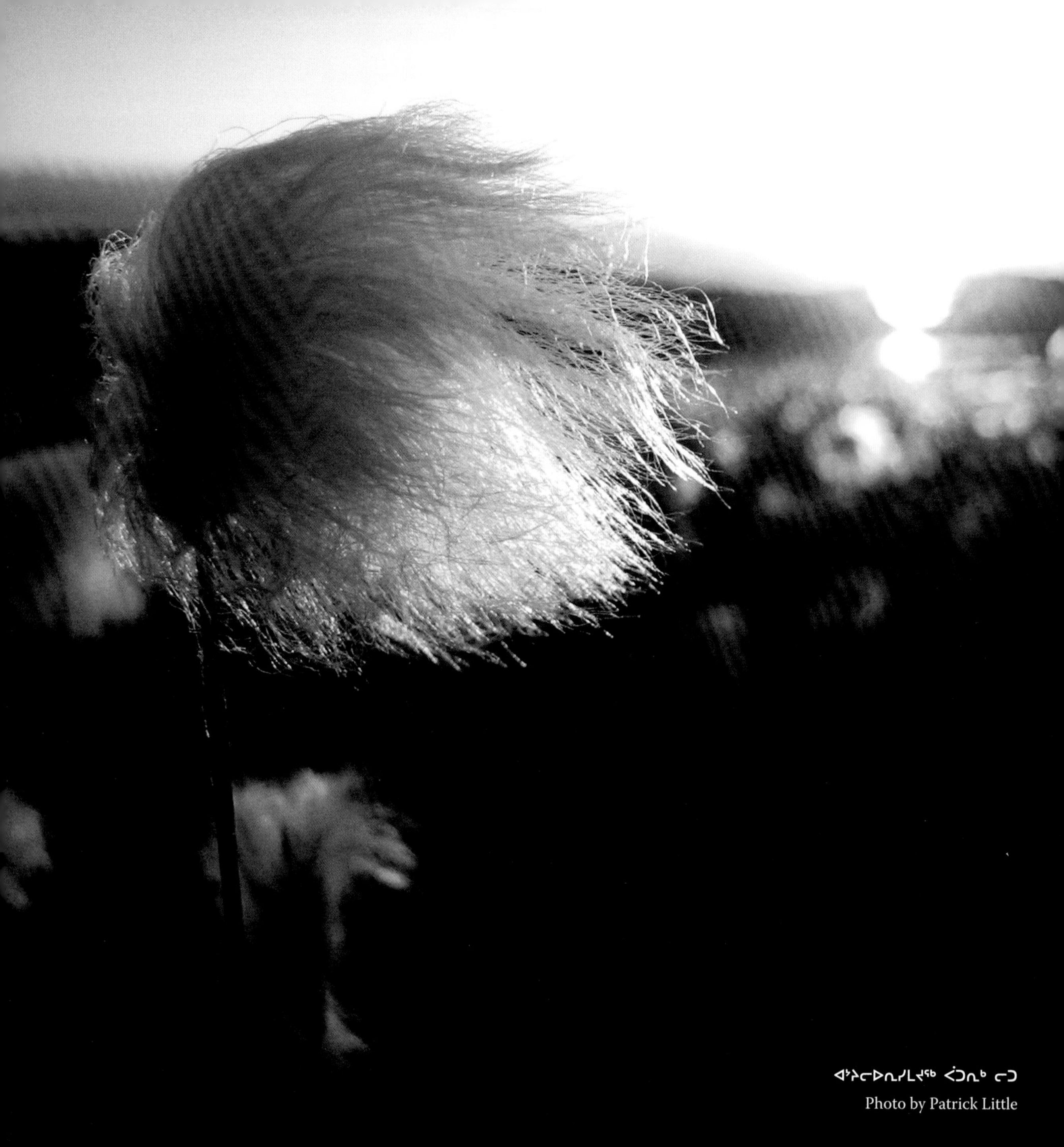

ᐊᔾᔨᓕᐅᕆᓯᒪᔪᖅ ᐹᑐᕆᒃ ᓕᑐ
Photo by Patrick Little

ᐳᐊᓗᙳᐊᑦ
Pualunnguat / Arctic Cotton

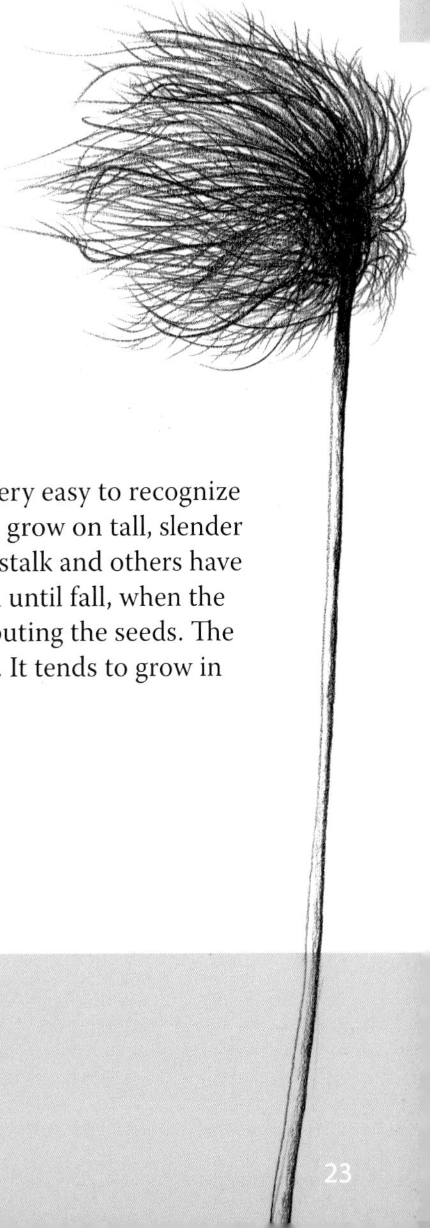

ᐳᐊᓗᙳᐊᑦ ᓄᓇᕗᒻᒥᑦ ᓇᒥᑐᐃᓐᓇᖅ ᓇᓂᔭᐅᔪᓐᓇᖅᑐᑦ. ᐃᓕᓴᕆᔭᕐᓂᖅᑐᐃᑦ ᐱᕈᕇᖅᓯᒪᑎᓪᓗᒋᑦ ᐱᕈᖅᓯᐊᖏᑦ ᖃᒃᑯᑑᒻᒪᑕ ᑕᑭᔪᓂᑦ ᐱᕈᕝᕕᖃᖅᑐᑎᒃ, ᐊᒥᑦᑐᑯᑖᑯᓗᓐᓂᑦ. ᐳᐊᓗᙳᐊᑦ ᐊᔾᔨᒌᖏᑦᑑᑕᐅᒻᒪᑕ ᐃᓚᖏᑦ ᐳᐊᓗᙳᐊᖃᖃᑦᑕᖅᑐᑦ ᐊᑕᐅᓯᕐᒥᑦ ᐃᓚᖏᓪᓗ ᐊᒥᓲᓂᖅᓴᓂᑦ. ᐱᕈᕇᖃᑦᑕᖅᑐᑦ ᐊᐅᔭᕋᑖᒃᑯᑦ ᐅᑭᐊᒃᓴᕋᓱᓐᓂᖓᓂᑦ, ᑎᑦᑕᐅᓇᓱᓐᓂᖏᓐᓂᑦ ᐱᕈᖅᓯᐊᒃᓴᖏᑦ, ᓯᐊᒻᒪᒃᑐᑎᒃ. ᐱᕈᕝᕕᖏᑦ ᑕᑭᓂᖃᕈᓐᓇᖅᑐᑦ 15–30 ᓯᐊᓐᑎᒦᑐᓂᑦ. ᑲᑎᒻᒪᒃᑯᔪᐃᑦ, ᐊᒻᒪᓗ ᒪᓴᕈᔪᒻᒦᒃᑯᔪᐃᑦ ᓄᓇᔭᒥᑦ.

Pualunnguat (Arctic cotton) is found across Nunavut. It is very easy to recognize when it is in bloom—its blossoms are bright white puffs that grow on tall, slender stalks. Some varieties of pualunnguat have one blossom per stalk and others have several. Its blossoms appear early in the summer and remain until fall, when the silky strands of the puffs are blown away on the wind, distributing the seeds. The stalks of pualunnguat grow from about 15 cm to 30 cm high. It tends to grow in large patches, usually across wetter parts of the tundra.

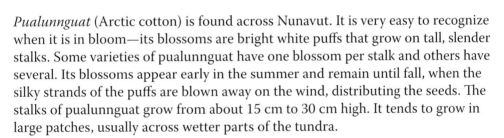

ᐳᐊᓗᙳᐊᑦ ᐊᑐᖅᑕᐅᒐᔪᑦ ᒪᓂᒃᓴᐅᓪᓗᑎᑦ ᖁᓪᓕᕐᒧᑦ. ᒪᓂᓕᐅᕐᓗᓂ ᐃᑯᐊᓚᑦᑎᐊᕐᓂᐊᖅᑐᒥᒃ ᐊᑯᓂᒃᑯᑦ, ᐳᐊᓗᙳᐊᑦ ᒥᖅᑯᖏᓐᓂᑦ ᒪᓂᕐᒧᑦ ᐃᓚᓕᐅᔾᔨᓗᑎᑦ ᓇᓕᒧᕇᑦᑐᑎᑦ (ᒪᓂᖅ; p. 29). ᑲᑎᑦᑐᒋᑦ ᐳᐊᓗᙳᐊᑦ ᒪᓂᕐᓗ ᐊᒃᓴᓕᑦᑐᒋᑦ ᐊᒡᒐᓐᓄᑦ ᑲᑎᑦᑎᐊᕐᓂᐊᕐᒪᑕ. ᐱᑕᖅᑲᖅᑎᓐᓇᒋᑦᓕ ᒪᓂᖅ ᐳᐊᓗᙳᐊᑦᓗ, ᐃᓇᖏᖅᑕᐅᔪᓐᓇᖅᑐᑦ ᓱᐳᑎᓄᑦ (p. 33). ᑕᐃᒪᑦᑕᐅ ᐊᑐᕋᒃᓴᐅᒐᓗᐊᖅ ᐅᕐᔪ (p. 99), ᑭᓯᐊᓂ ᐱᐅᒋᔭᐅᖏᓐᓂᖅᓴᐃᑦ ᐃᑭᑦᑐᑎᒃ ᓄᖑᓴᕋᐃᓗᐊᕐᒪᑕ.

The main use of pualunnguat is as the wick of a *qulliq* (soapstone lamp). To make a wick that will burn evenly and last long, use the silky strands of pualunnguat with an equal amount of *maniq* (lamp moss; p. 29). Roll the pualunnguat and maniq between your palms to combine them. When maniq or pualunnguat is unavailable, either can be substituted with *suputit* (see *uqpi suputillu,* Arctic willow; p. 33). Another possible substitution is *urju* (peat moss; p. 99), but this is not preferred because urju burns too quickly.

ᐳᐊᓗᙳᐊᑦ ᐊᒥᓱᓂᑦ ᐊᑑᑎᓕ ᓴᓗᒻᒪᖅᓴᐃᔭᑎᑦᑎᐊᕙᐅᑦᑐᓂᓗ ᐊᑲᐅᓯᓴᐅᑎᖄᕐᔪᑦᑐᑦᓂᓗ. ᐋᓚᓯᓕ ᐃᖅᑲᐅᒪᒍᖅ ᓄᑕᕋᖕᒋᑕ ᖃᓚᓯᖕᒋᓐᓄᑦ ᓴᓗᒻᒪᖅᓴᐃᔾᔪᑎᒋᖅᑲᑦᑕᓚᐅᖅᓯᒪᒐᒥᐅ. ᓄᑕᕋᖅ ᐃᓅᕋᑖᖅᑎᑦᓗᒍ, ᖃᓚᓯᖕᒐ ᒪᒥᒐᓱᐊᕐᓂᖕᒐᓂᑦ ᒪᕿᕈᔪᓰᕌᓗᒻᒪᑕ. ᐳᐊᓗᙳᐊᖅ ᐅᓐᓄᐊᓕᒫᖅ ᐃᓕᓯᒪᒍᓂ, ᒪᕿᕈᔪᒃᑐᓂ ᓴᓗᐊᖅᑎᑦᑎᒻᒪᑦ

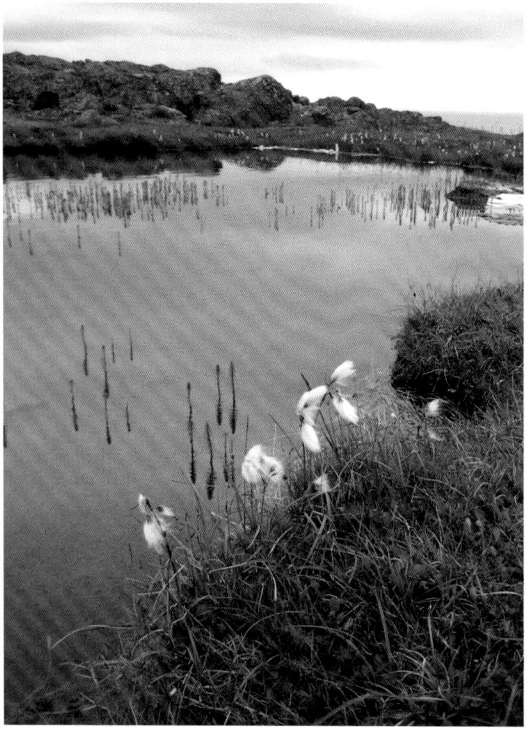

ᐳᐊᓗᙳᐊᑦ ᑕᓯᐅᑉ ᑭᑦᓕᖓᓂ ᓂᐊᖁᙴᒥᑦ.

Pualunnguat at the edge of a pond in Niaqunnguuq (Apex).

ᓴᓗᒻᒪᕐᒃᓴᐃᔾᔨᑎᑦᑎᐊᕙᐅᓪᓗᓂ. ᑕᐃᒫᑦᑕᐅ, ᐳᐊᓗᙳᐊᑦ ᐊᑐᕋᒃᓴᐅᕗᑦ ᓱᐅᓯᓂᔪᒧᑦ ᐃᓐᓇᕐᒧᑦ ᓱᕈᓯᕐᒧᓐᓂᑦ. ᓱᐅᑎ ᒪᕐᑭᒍᓂ, ᐳᐊᓗᙳᐊᑦ ᑕᐳᑦᑖ ᐊᑐᕋᒃᓴᐅᔪᕐᒃ ᐱᕈᕐᕕᖕᒐ ᑕᒪᓐᓇ ᐊᑕᐅᓂ, ᓲᕐᑐᓕ ᓱᐅᑎᓕᓇᔾᔨᑎᑐᑦ. ᐳᐊᓗᙳᐊᑦ ᓴᓗᒻᒪᕐᒃᓴᐃᔾᔨᑕᐅᔪᓐᓇᕐᒥᔪᑦ ᑭᓕᕐᒃᑐᒧᑦ ᒪᑦᑐᑎᕐᒃᑕᐅᓚᐅᙱᑎᓪᓗᒍ ᓯᓕ. ᐳᐊᓗᙳᐊᑦ ᑲᒥᐅᑉ ᐊᑯᓐᓂᖕᒐᓃᑦᑎᑕᐅᕐᒃᑦᑕᕐᒃᑐᕕᓃᑦ ᐊᑐᐃᓐᓇᐅᒐᔭᕐᒪᑕ ᐊᑐᕐᒃᑕᐅᒥᐊᕐᒃᑲᓕᕈᑎ.

Pualunnguat has many uses as a general cleaning cloth with mild medicinal properties. Aalasi recalls using it to clean the umbilical cords of her babies. After a baby is born, there may be some secretion from the cord before it heals. If the pualunnguat is left on overnight, it will absorb any secretion, and it will keep the area clean. Similarly, pualunnguat can be used to clean ear infections in adults and children. If there is any leakage from the ear, use a puff of pualunnguat with the stem still attached, like a cotton swab. Pualunnguat can also be used to clean wounds before they are mended. People kept puffs of pualunnguat folded into the liners of their *kamiit* (sealskin boots) for easy access whenever it was needed.

ᐋᓚᓯ ᐃᕐᒃᑲᐅᒪᔪᕐᒃ ᐊᖕᒐᔪᕐᒃᑳᖕᒋᒃ ᓄᐊᑦᑎᕐᒃᑦᑕᕐᓂᕐᒪᑎᒃ ᐳᐊᓗᙳᐊᓂᑦ ᐊᑭᓯᓚᐊᓇᔭᐅᓂᐊᕐᒥᒃ ᕐᑲᓂᒪᔪᒧᑦ. ᓂᕈᒥᓐᓂᑯᓗᖕᒋᑦ ᐊᑲᐅᓯᔾᔨᑕᐅᔪᓐᓇᕐᒪᑕ ᐊᑲᐅᑦᑎᐊᖕᒋᑦᑐᒧᑦ, ᐱᓗᐊᕐᒃᑐᑎᒃ ᓂᐊᕐᑯᙳᔪᓄᑦ. ᒥᕐᒃᑯᖕᒋᑦᑕᐅ ᐅᕐᒃᑰᔪᑯᓗᓐᓂᑦ ᐊᓪᓕᓂᓕᐊᖑᔪᓐᓇᕐᒥᔪᑦ ᐃᓅᕐᑖᕐᒧᑦ ᐊᑐᕐᒃᑕᐅᓂᐊᕐᓗᓂ. ᒥᕐᒃᑯᖕᒋᑦ ᕐᑲᓪᓗᓅᕐᒃᑕᐅ ᐊᑯᓐᓂᖕᒐᓄᑦ ᒥᕐᒃᓲᕐᒃᑕᐅᓗᑎᑦ ᓅᕈᓘᔭᕈᓐᓇᐃᓕᒐᔭᕐᒃᑐᑦ. ᑕᐃᒫ ᓴᓇᓗᒍ, ᐳᐊᓗᓄᑦ ᑲᒥᓐᓄᓘᓐᓃᑦ ᐃᓗᓪᓕᓕᐊᖑᔪᓐᓇᕐᒃᑐᑦ.

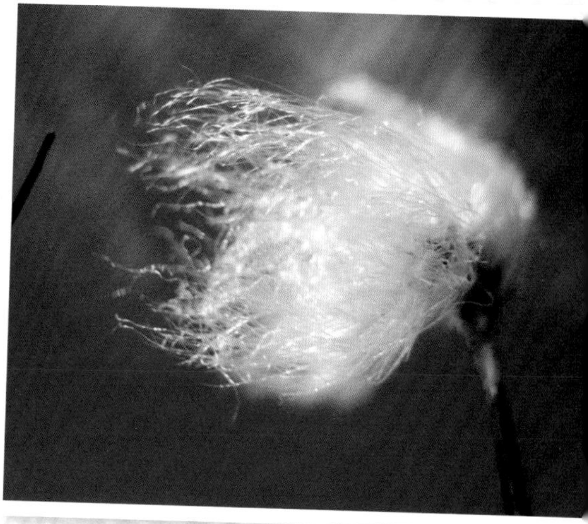

ᓄᓇᔭᒥᑦ ᑕᑯᔭᕐᓂᕐᒃᑐᑯᓗᐃᑦ ᐳᐊᓗᙳᐊᑦ ᕐᑲᑯᕐᒃᑕᐃᑦ ᒥᕐᒃᑯᖕᒋᑦ.

The white puffs of pualunnguat are easy to spot across the tundra.

Aalasi recalls her parents collecting pualunnguat to make a pillow for someone who was sick. The silky strands have gentle healing properties that help with any ailment, but especially with headaches. The puffs can also be used to make a soothing and insulating mattress for an infant. The puffs can be loosely quilted between two layers of cloth to keep them in place. In this same way, this plant can also be used as a liner for mittens or kamiit.

ᐳᐊᓗᙳᐊᑦ ᓄᐊᓐᓂᐊᕐᓗᒋᑦ ᐱᐅᓛᖑᕗᖅ ᐊᐅᔭᕐᑲᐅᓕᖅᑎᓪᓗᒍ ᒥᖅᑯᒃᑭᑦᑎᐊᕙᓗᑎᓪᓗᒋᑦ. ᑭᓯᐊᓂ, ᐊᑐᓇᐊᕐᑲᕐᒪᑕ ᓯᕗᓂᐊᒍᑦ ᓄᐊᒐᒃᓴᑦᑎᐊᖑᒻᒥᔪᑦ. ᓄᐊᑕᐅᓯᒪᓕᖅᑎᓪᓗᒋᓪᓕ ᐳᐊᓗᙳᐊᑦ ᒥᖅᑯᖏᑦ, ᐅᑭᐅᓕᒫᕐᒧᑦ ᐊᑐᖅᓴᐃᑦ. ᓄᐊᓯᒪᔪᑦ ᐳᐊᓗᙳᐊᑦ ᐆᒪᑯᑖᑦᑎᑕᒃᓴᐅᒻᒥᔪᑦ ᐹᖅᓯᒪᓗᒋᑦ ᐃᒻᒫᕐᔪᒃᓯᒪᓗᒋᓪᓗ.

The best time to collect pualunnguat is in the late summer when the plant is very fluffy. But, if necessary, it can be collected earlier. Once the puffs of pualunnguat have been collected, they can be kept and used all winter. The puffy blossoms and stalks can also be kept alive for a long time if they are placed in a tin or bucket with a small amount of water at the bottom.

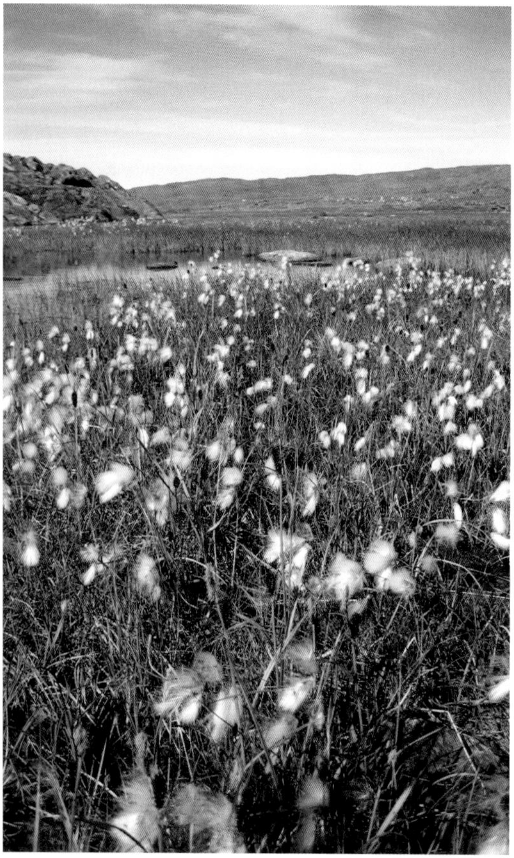

ᐃᕐᑲᓗᐃᑦ ᑰᖓᓂ ᐳᐊᓗᙳᐊᑦ ᐊᒥᓱᐃᑦ (ᓱᐅᓪᕕᐊ ᒍᓇᓂᐅᓪ).

A marsh of pualunnguat near Iqaluit Kuunga (the Sylvia Grinnell River).

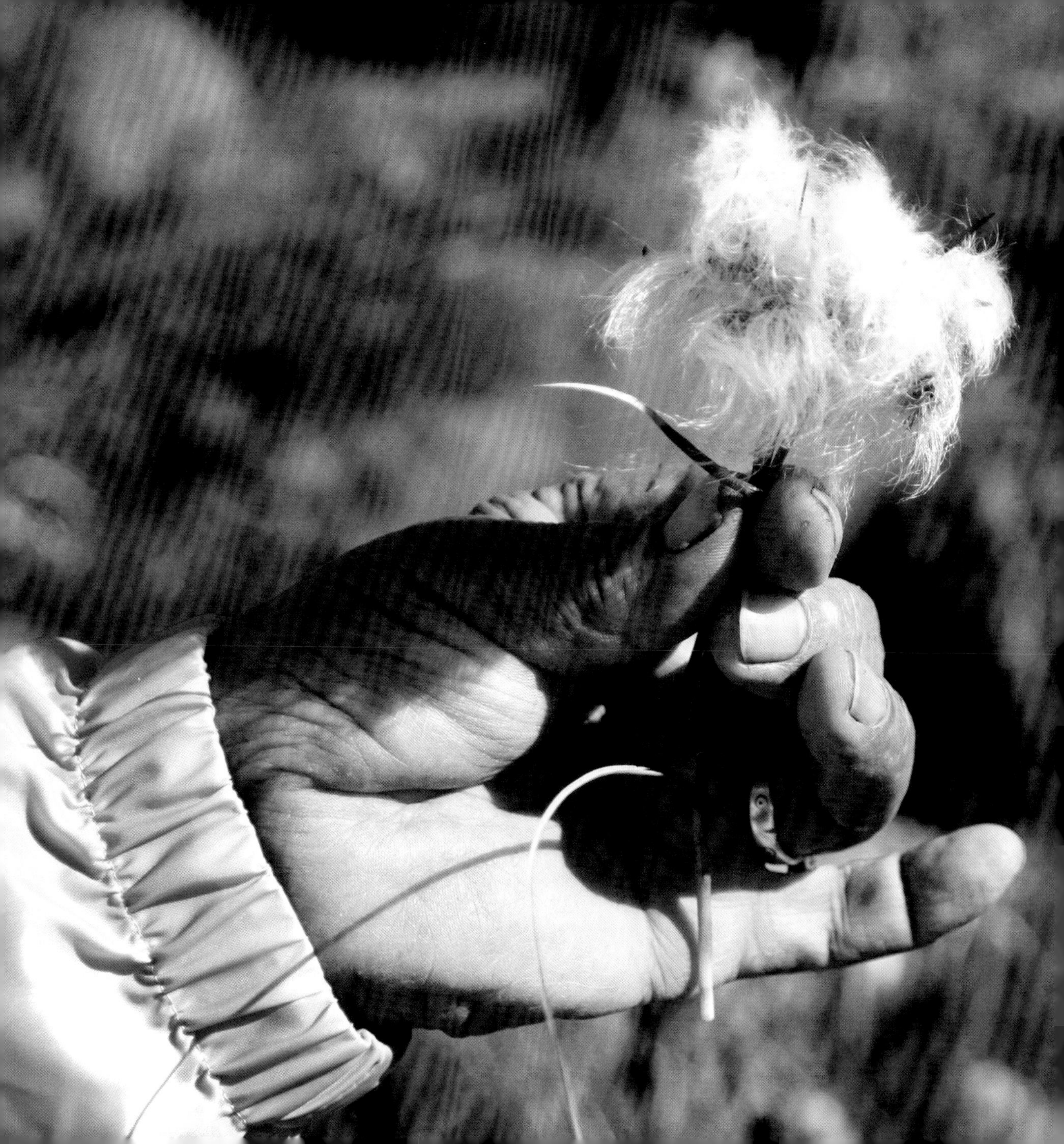

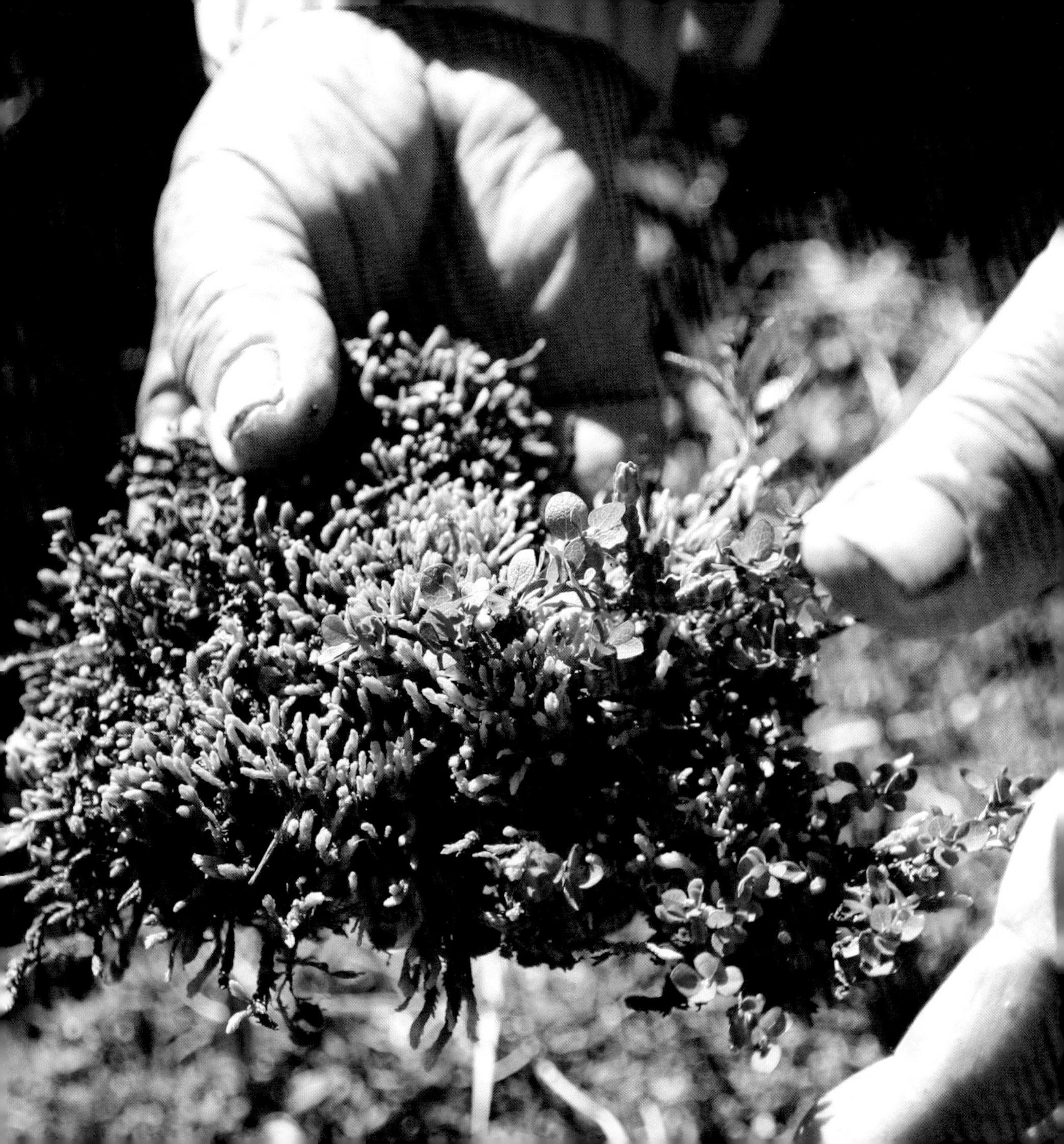

ᒪᓂᖅ

Maniq / Lamp Moss

ᒪᓂᖅ ᐱᕈᕐᓂᖅᓴᐅᖃᑦᑕᖅᑐᑦ ᓄᓇᕗᒻᒥᑦ ᐅᖅᑰᓂᖅᓴᓂᑦ ᐊᑦᑎᓐᓂᖅᓴᒥᑦ, ᐱᑕᖃᙱᓐᓂᖅᓴᐅᓪᓗᓂ ᖁᑦᑎᓐᓂᖅᓴᒥᑦ. ᒥᑭᑦᑐᑯᓘᓪᓗᑎᑦ ᑲᑎᒻᒪᔪᕕᔾᔪᐊᑯᓘᓪᓗᑎᑦ ᐱᕈᖃᑦᑕᖅᑐᑦ ᖃᐅᓯᐅᓪᓗᑎᓪᓗ.

Maniq (lamp moss) is a moss that is common in the more southern parts of Nunavut and less common in the High Arctic. It grows as a moist, spongy carpet made up of very small mounds.

ᐊᑑᑎᓪᓗᐊᙵ ᒪᓂᐅᑉ ᓇᓕᒧᙵᓂᑦ ᑲᑎᑦᑎᓗᓂ ᐳᐊᓗᙳᐊᒧᑦ (p. 23) ᐅᕝᕙᓘᓐᓃᑦ ᓱᐳᑎᒧᑦ (ᐅᖅᐲᑦ ᓱᐳᑎᓪᓗ; p. 33) ᖁᓪᓕᕐᒧᑦ ᒪᓂᐅᓂᐊᕐᓗᑎᑦ. ᐳᐊᓗᙳᐊᑦ ᓱᐳᑎᓪᓗ ᐱᑕᖃᙱᑉᐳᑎᑦ, ᒪᓂᖅ ᑲᑎᑕᒃᓴᐅᕙᑦ ᐅᕐᔪᓄᑦ (ᐅᕐᔪ; p. 99) ᒪᓂᓕᐊᓇᓗᒋᑦ, ᑭᓯᐊᓂ ᐅᕐᔪ ᒪᓂᔅᓴᒧᑦ ᐃᓚᓕᐅᑎᓯᒪᓗᒍ ᓱᒃᑲᓂᖅᓴᒥᑦ ᐃᑭᒃᑲᔭᖅᑐᖅ ᐳᐊᓗᙳᐊᑦ ᓱᐳᑎᐅᓪᓘᓐᓃᑦ ᓴᓂᐊᓂ, ᑕᐃᒪ ᐊᑐᕈᒥᓇᙱᓐᓂᖅᓴᐅᔾᔪᑎᒋᕚ.

The main use of maniq is to combine it in equal parts with either *pualunnguat* (Arctic cotton; p. 23) or *suputit* (*uqpi suputillu*, Arctic willow; p. 33) to make a wick for a qulliq. If neither pualunnguat nor suputit is available, maniq can also be combined with *urju* (peat moss; p. 99) to make a wick, but a wick made with urju will burn more quickly than a wick made of pualunnguat or suputit, so it is less desirable.

ᒪᓂᖅ ᔫᕈᓗᒃᑐᒧᑦ ᐊᑲᐅᓯᔾᔪᑕᐅᔪᓐᓇᕐᒥᔪᖅ ᐅᖅᓯᐃᔭᐃᒻᒪᑦ. ᔫᕈᓗᒃᑐᖅ, ᓂᕆᔪᓐᓇᖅᑐᖅ (ᑑ ᑖᓕᑎᑐᑦ ᐊᖏᑎᒋᔭᒥᑦ). ᑕᒧᐊᑦᑕᐃᓕᓗᒍ. ᐸᓚᐅᒫᕐᒥᑦ ᓂᕆᖅᑲᓯᐅᔾᔨᖅᑯᔭᖅ ᐄᔭᕐᓂᕐᓂᖅᓴᐅᓂᐊᕐᒪᑦ.

Maniq can also be used to help with heartburn, as it absorbs the excess fat in the stomach causing the heartburn. To treat heartburn, swallow a small bunch (about the size of a toonie). Do not chew it. If necessary, combine it with bannock to make it easier to swallow.

ᐋᓚᓯ ᐃᖅᑲᐅᒪᔪᖅ ᒪᓂᖅ ᐊᑐᖅᑕᐅᖃᑦᑕᓚᐅᕐᓂᖏᓐᓂᑦ ᖃᒧᑎᐅᑉ ᐱᕐᖀᖏᓐᓄᑦ ᐱᐊᒃᓴᐅᑎᓕᐅᖅᑐᓄᑦ ᓂᓚᒻᒥᑦ. ᐃᖅᑲᐅᒪᑦᑎᐊᖅᑐᖅ ᐊᑖᑕᖓ ᖃᒧᑎᒥᓂᑦ ᐱᐊᒃᓴᐃᑎᓪᓗᒍ ᒪᓂᖅ ᖃᐅᓯᖅ ᖃᒧᑎᐅ ᐱᕐᖀᖏᓐᓄᑦ ᐊᑦᑐᖅᑕᖅᑎᖕᖓᓗᒃᑐᓂᐅᒃ.

Aalasi also recalls that maniq can be used as a sponge to put a new layer of ice on a dogsled runner. She recalls her father working on their sled runners and the quiet rush of the wet maniq passing along them.

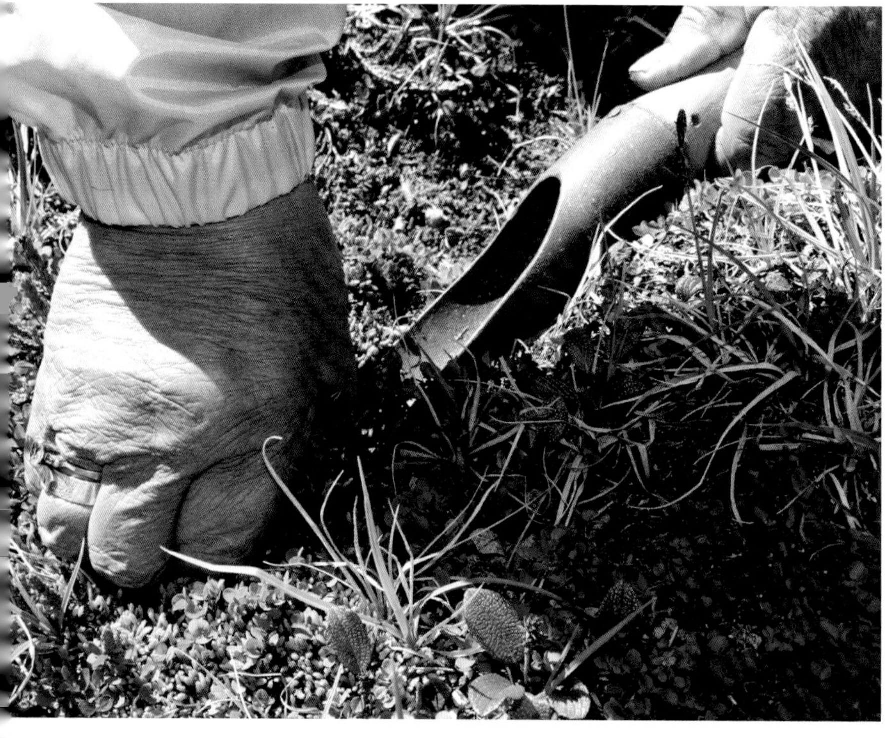

ᐋᓚᓯ ᒪᓂᖅᓂᑦ ᐲᖅᓯᔪᖅ ᐃᖅᑲᓗᐃᑦ ᑰᖓᑕ ᓴᓂᐊᓂᑦ (ᓯᐅᓪᕕᐊ ᒍᕆᓂᐅᓪ).

Aalasi scoops up a mound of maniq near Iqaluit Kunnga (the Sylvia Grinnell River).

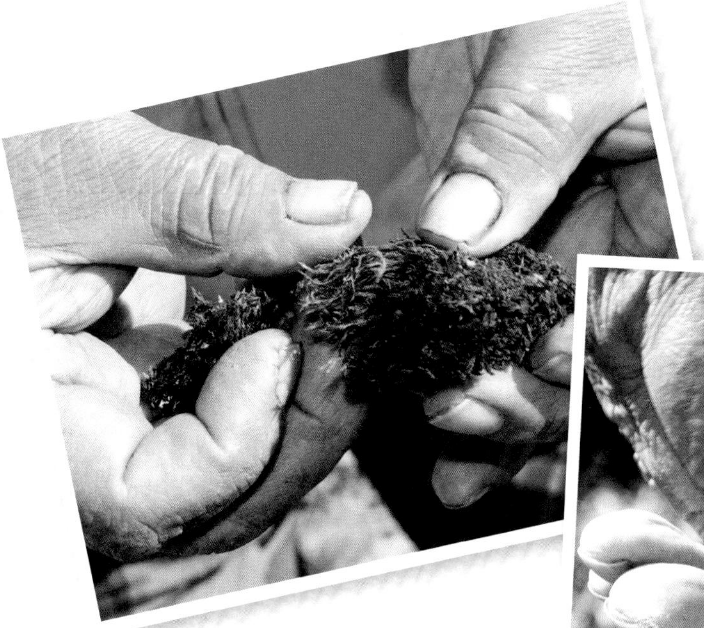

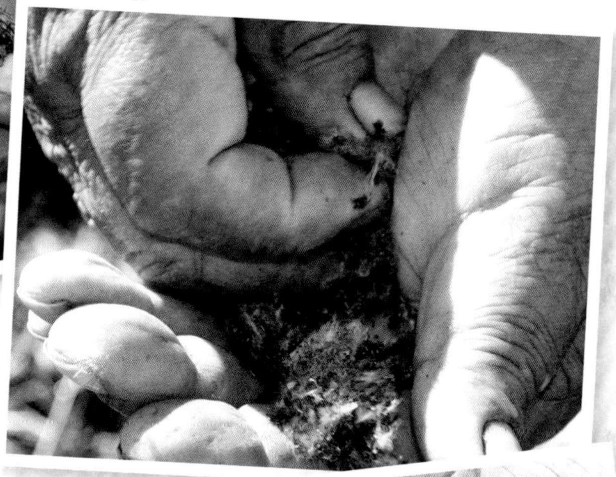

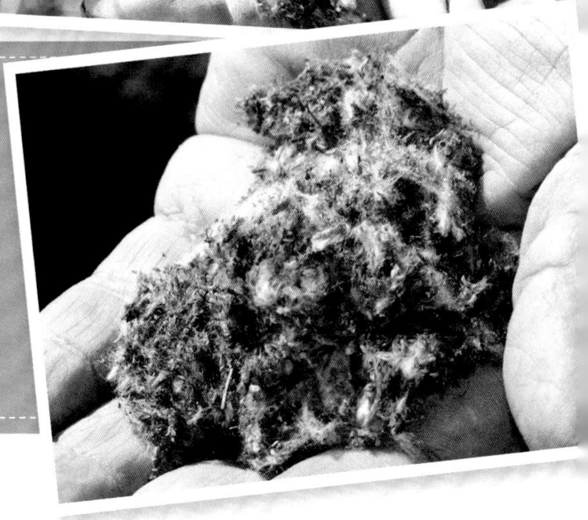

ᐋᓚᓯᐅᑉ ᓱᕋᑦᑎᖅᑕᖓ ᒪᓂᖅ ᐃᓚᓕᐅᑎᓂᐊᕋᒥᐅ
ᐳᐊᓗᙳᐊᓄᑦ, ᐃᑯᐊᓚᑦᑎᐊᓲᕐᒥᑦ ᓄᖑᓴᕋᐃᖏᑦᑐᒥᒃ
ᒪᓂᔅᓴᓕᐅᖅᑐᖅ. ᒪᓂᖅ ᖁᓪᓕᕐᒧᑦ ᒪᓂᔅᓴᐅᒡᒍᔪᑦ,
ᑭᓯᐊᓂᑦᑕᐅ ᐊᑐᕋᒃᓴᐃᑦ ᓲᕈᓗᓗᐊᖅᑐᒧᑦ ᓂᕆᔭᐅᓗᑎᑦ.

Aalasi breaks maniq apart to combine it with a handful of pualunnguat, preparing an ideal mixture for a slow-burning qulliq wick. Maniq is primarily used as a wick for a qulliq, but it can also help with heartburn when swallowed.

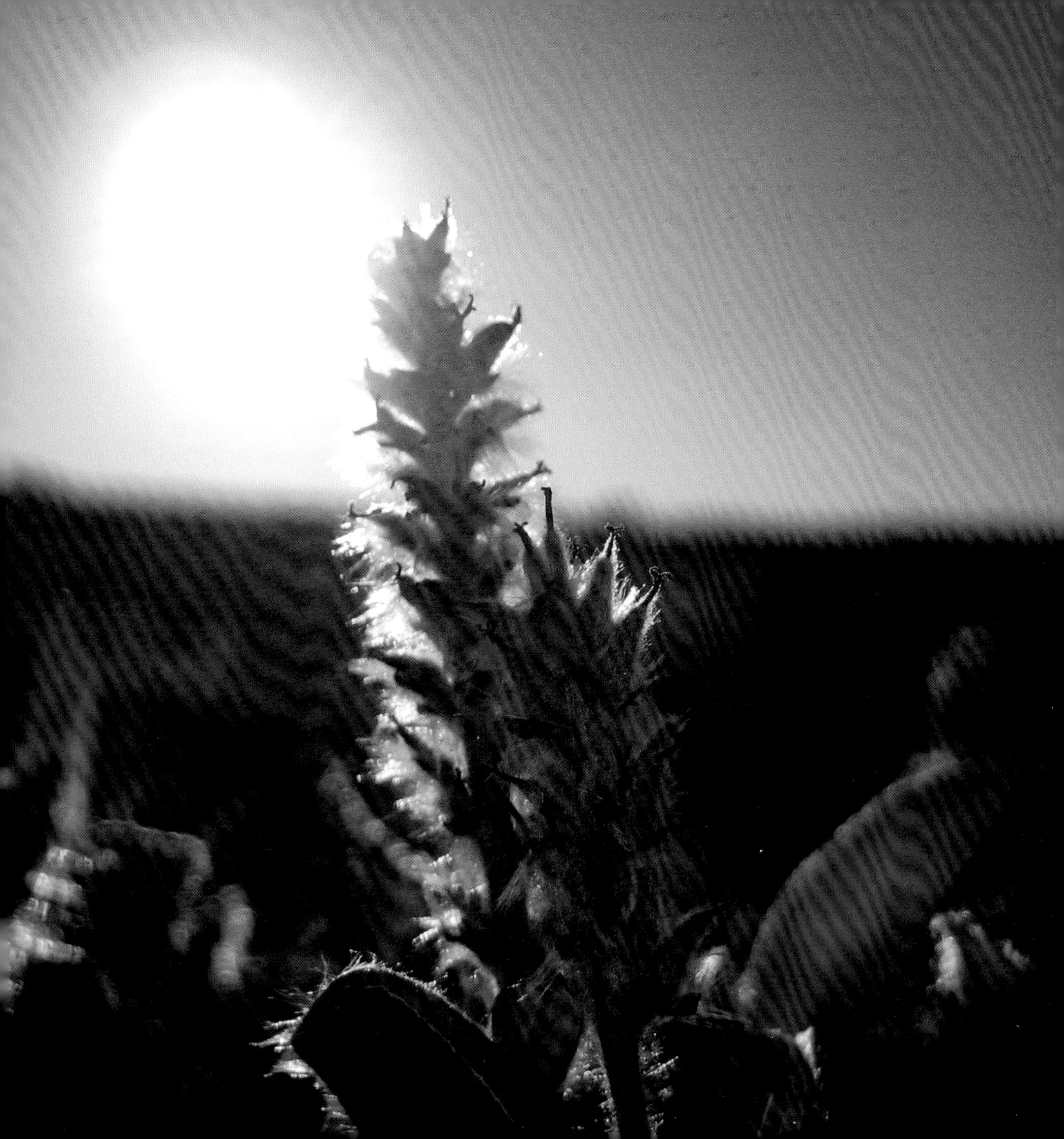

ᐅᖅᐱ ᓱᐳᑎᓪᓗ
Uqpi Suputillu / Arctic Willow

ᓱᐳᑎᑦ ᖃᑯᖅᑕᐅᓂᑯᓗᒋᕙᐃᑦ ᐱᓇᖅᑰᑉ ᐱᕈᖅᑲᑦᑕᖅᑐ ᐅᐱᕐᖕᒫᖖᒍᕋᑖᖅᑎᓪᓗᒍ. ᐅᖅᐱᐅᓂᖕᒐᓕ ᓇᑲᒋᕚ. ᑖᓐᓇ ᑎᑎᕋᖅᓯᒪᔫᑉ ᐊᑎᖕᒐ ᐅᖅᐱ ᓱᐳᑎᓪᓘᕗᑦ ᐱᔾᔪᑎᒋᓪᓗᒍ ᐊᑐᓂ ᐅᖃᐅᓯᐅᓂᐊᖅᒪᑏᒃ. ᐱᕈᖅᑰᑉ ᐃᓚᐃᓐᓇᖕᒐ ᑕᐃᔭᐅᒡᒍᔪᖅ ᐅᖃᐅᓯᐅᑎᓪᓗᒋᑦ ᐱᔾᔪᑎᒋᓪᓗᒍ ᐱᕈᖅᑰᑉ ᐃᓚᐃᓐᓇᑐᐊᖕᒐ ᐅᖃᐅᑕᐅᕙᒻᒪᑦ.

Suputit is the fluffy white part of this plant that appears on the catkin early in the summer. *Uqpi* is the woody stem part of the plant. This plant chapter is called *Uqpi Suputillu* ("Uqpi and Suputit") because both parts of the plant will be discussed together. The words are often used separately to refer to the plant's specific parts.

ᐅᖅᐱ ᓱᐳᑎᓪᓗ ᓄᓇᕗᓚᒫᐸᓗᒻᒥᑦ ᐱᑕᖅᓲᑦ. ᐱᕈᖅᓯᐊᖕᒋᑦ ᐊᖕᒋᑦᓗᑎᑦ ᐊᐅᐸᕈᔪᑦᑐᑦ ᐊᒻᒪ ᑐᖑᔪᖅᑐᑎᑦ ᐊᐅᔭᓖᑲᒃᑯᑦ ᐱᕈᖅᐸᑦᑐᑎᒃ. ᐱᕈᖅᓯᐊᒃᓴᖅᑲᓚᖀᖕᒐᒥᑦ ᖃᑯᖅᑖᑯᓗᒻᒥᑦ ᒥᖅᑯᖅᑲᓚᖅᑲᑦᑕᖅᑐᑦ (ᓱᐳᑎᑦ). ᐅᖃᐅᔭᖕᒋᑦ ᕿᑦᓚᖅᑐᑎᑦ ᑐᖑᑦᑐᓇᑦᑐᑎᑦ. ᓵᑦᑐᑯᓗᐃᑦ, ᑭᑦᓚᖕᒋᑦ ᑐᑭᓚᐊᑦᑎᐊᖅᑐᑎᑦ ᐊᒻᒪ ᕿᑎᖕᒐᓄ ᐃᒧᕈᔪᕆᐊᖅᓯᒪᖅᑰᔭᑦᓗᑎᑦ. ᖁᖅᓱᖅᑰᓚᖅᑲᑦᑕᖅᑐᑦ ᐅᑭᐊᒃᓵᒃᑯᑦ. ᕿᔫᓂᖓ (ᐅᖅᐱ) ᑲᔫᔪᑦ. ᑖᓐᓇ ᓄᓇᕋᖅ ᐊᖕᒋᓂᖅᑲᕈᓐᓇᖅᑐ 3–25 ᓴᐊᓐᑎᒦᑐᒥᑦ. ᓄᓇᒃᑰᖕᒐᖅᑲᑦᑕᖅᑐᑦ ᐱᕈᖅᓂᖕᒋᑦ ᑭᓯᐊᓂᑦᑕᐅ ᐃᓚᖕᒋᑦ ᖁᒻᒧᑐᐃᓐᓇᖅ ᐱᕈᓲᑦ.

Uqpi suputillu is a common shrub in many parts of Nunavut.

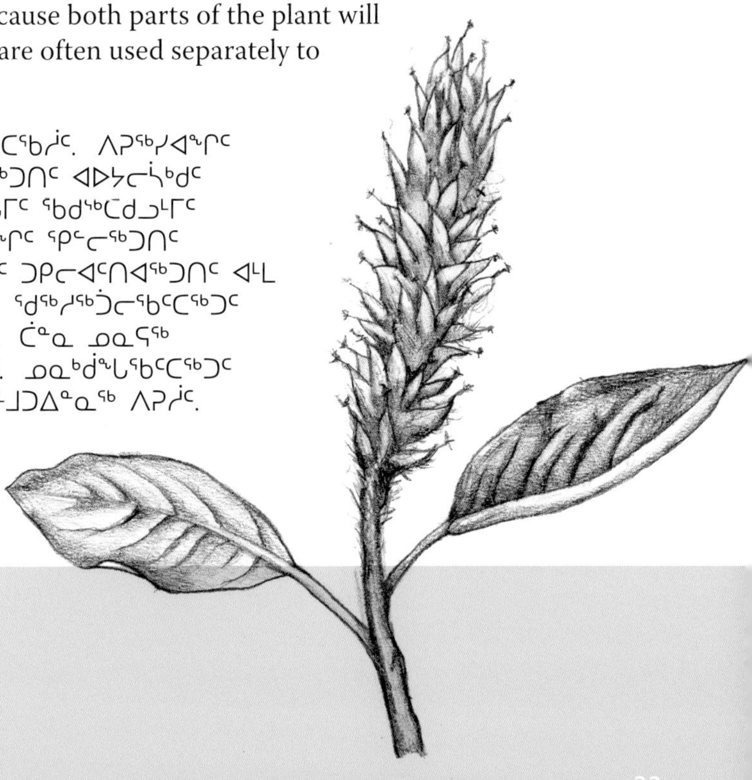

It has large pink and green catkins that bloom early in the summer. When the seeds begin to ripen, they are surrounded by soft white fluff (suputit). The leaves are shiny and bright green. They are thin, smooth-edged, and often curled slightly toward the centre. They turn bright yellow in the fall. The stems (uqpi) are woody and brown. This plant can grow from 3 cm to 25 cm high. It can grow along the ground or vertically, toward the sky.

ᐅᖅᐱ, ᓇᑲᐅᓂᓇᖒ ᐊᑑᑎᖅᑲᖅᑐᖅ ᐊᔾᔩᖕᒋᑦᑐᓄᑦ. ᐃᑭᑕᐅᔪᓐᓇᖅᑐᑦ (ᑎᐱᑦᑎᐊᓇᑦᑐᑯᓘᑦᑐᑎᒃ). ᐊᑕᐅᓯᑯᑖᒃ ᐃᒐᕝᔪᑕᐅᔪᓐᓇᖅᑐ ᐃᑯᒪᒥᑦ ᐊᐅᓚᑦᑎᕝᔪᑎᒋᔭᐅᓗᓂ. ᑲᑎᖅᓱᖅᓗᒋᑦ ᓇᑲᖕᒋᑦ ᐊᓗᖅᓗᐃᔭᐅᑎᓕᐊᓇᔭᒃᓴᐅᒻᒥᔪᑦ ᐊᒻᒪ ᐊᑦᓚᓂᓚᐊᓇᔭᒃᓴᐅᒋᑦᓗᑎᒃ ᕿᓚᒃᓱᖅᓗᒋᑦ ᐊᑦᑐᓈᖅᓄᑦ ᐊᒥᕕᓂᖅᓄᑦᑑᓐᓃᑦ.

Uqpi, the woody stem part of the plant, can be used for many things. The small branches can be burned for fire (with a lovely scent). A single branch can be used to stir or control a fire as well. The branches can also be woven into entrance mats and sleeping pads when tied together with thread or pieces of skin.

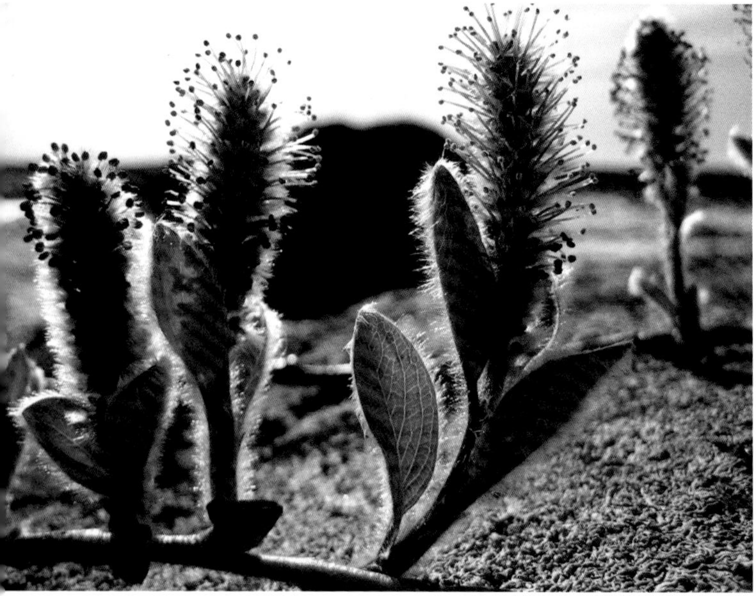

ᐊᐅᔭᖃᑖᖅ ᐱᕈᖅᑐᖕᒋᑦ ᐱᕈᖅᓯᒪᓕᖅᑎᑦᓗᒋᑦ.

New catkins of uqpi suputillu at the beginning of summer.

ᐊᐃᕋᖕᒋᑦ ᑕᒧᐊᔭᐅᔪᓐᓇᖅᑐᑦ ᑭᒍᓯᓇᔪᒧᑦ ᐱᔪᓐᓃᕐᓂᐊᕐᒪᑦ. ᐃᑉᐱᓐᓂᐊᔪᓐᓃᕈᑎᖄᕐᔪᒻᒪᑕ. ᐃᐱᓐᓂᐊᔪᓐᓃᕈᑎ ᐊᑐᕈᒪᓗᒍ, ᖄᖕᒐ ᐊᐃᕋᖕᒐᑕ ᐲᔭᕐᓗᒍ ᑕᒧᐊᖁᔪᖅ ᐃᒃᓵᕿᓂᐊᕐᒪᑦ. ᐊᒻᒪᓗᑦᑕᐅ, ᐅᖃᐅᔭᖕᒋᑦ ᓂᕆᖁᔪᖅ, ᕿᔪᒃᓯᓐᓂᕈᔪᒃᑐᐃᑦ.

The roots can be chewed to relieve a toothache. They contain a mild anaesthetic. To access the anaesthetic, peel the root and chew on it to release the juices. Also, the leaves are edible. They have a mild, woody flavour.

ᓱᐳᑎᑦ, ᖃᑯᕐᓂᖕᒐ ᒥᖅᑯᕈᔪᑯᓗᒃ, ᐊᐅᔭᒃᑯᑦ ᓄᐊᑕᐅᓲᑦ, ᑎᑦᑕᐅᓚᐅᖕᒋᓐᓂᖕᒋᓐᓂᑦ. ᓱᐳᑎᑦ ᒪᓂᓕᐊᓇᔭᐅᒡᒍᔪᐃᑦ ᖁᑦᓕᕐᒧᑦ. ᒪᓂᓕᐊᖑᓂᐊᕐᓗᓂᓕ ᖁᑦᓕᕐᒧᑦ ᐊᑐᖅᑐᒃᓴᐅᓗᓂ, ᓱᐳᑎᑦ ᒪᓂᕐᒧᑦ ᑲᑎᑕᐅᒡᒍᔪᑦ ᓇᓕᒧᒦᑦᓗᐊᑐᐃᓐᓇᕐᓗᒋᑦ. ᐳᐊᓗᙳᐊᑦ (p. 29) ᒪᓂᕐᒧᑦ ᐃᓚᓕᐅᑎᔭᒃᓴᐅᒻᒥᔪᑦ ᒪᓂᓕᐊᖑᓂᐊᕐᓗᓂ. ᑭᓯᐊᓂ ᓱᐳᑎᑦ ᐱᐅᒋᔭᐅᓂᖅᓴᐅᓰᑦ ᓄᖕᒍᓴᕋᐃᖕᒋᓐᓂᖅᓴᐅᒻᒪᑕ. ᒪᓂᖅᑕᖃᖅᑎᓐᓇᒍᓕ, ᓱᐳᑎᑦ ᐃᓚᓕᐅᔾᔭᒃᓴᐅᕗᖅ ᐳᐊᓗᙳᐊᒧᑦ. ᐊᒻᒪᓯᓕ ᑕᐃᒪ ᐅᕐᔪ (p. 23) ᐊᑐᖕᒑᕋᒃᓴᑦᑎᐊᖅ (p. 99), ᑭᓯᐊᓂ ᐅᕐᔪ ᐊᑐᖅᑕᐅᖃᑦᑕᖅᑐᖅ ᐊᓯᒃᓴᖃᖕᒋᑦᑎᐊᖅᑎᓪᓗᒍ ᐱᔾᔪᑎᒋᓪᓗᒍ ᓄᖕᒍᓴᕋᐃᓐᓂᖕᒐ.

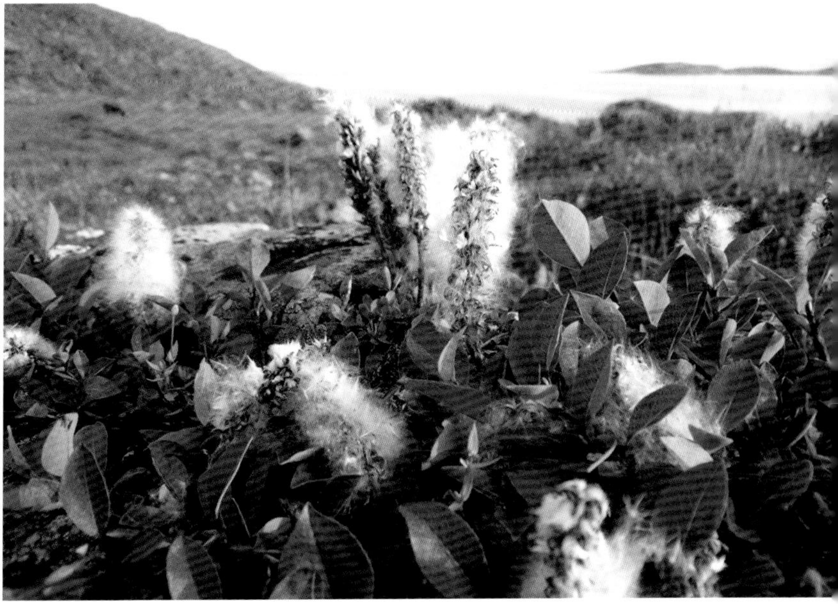

ᒥᖅᑯᓕᑯᓗᐃᑦ ᐊᐅᔭᓪᓗᐊᒃᑯᑦ, ᐃᖃᓗᐃᑦ ᐃᒪᖕᒐᓄᑦ ᓵᙵᒐᓪᓗᐊᖅᑐᑦ (ᐃᖃᓗᐃᑦ, ᓄᓇᕗᑦ).

Fuzzy suputit in mid-summer, overlooking Frobisher Bay (Iqaluit, Nunavut).

Suputit, the white fluffy part, is collected in the early summer, before it blows away. The main use of suputit is as the wick of a qulliq. To make the wick for a qulliq, suputit is usually mixed with *maniq* (lamp moss; p. 29) in equal parts. *Pualunnguat* (Arctic cotton; p. 23) can also be combined with maniq to make a wick. However, some prefer suputit because it burns slightly more slowly. When maniq is unavailable, suputit can be combined with pualunnguat. Another possible substitution is *urju* (peat moss; p. 99), but urju is only used when nothing else is available because it burns too quickly.

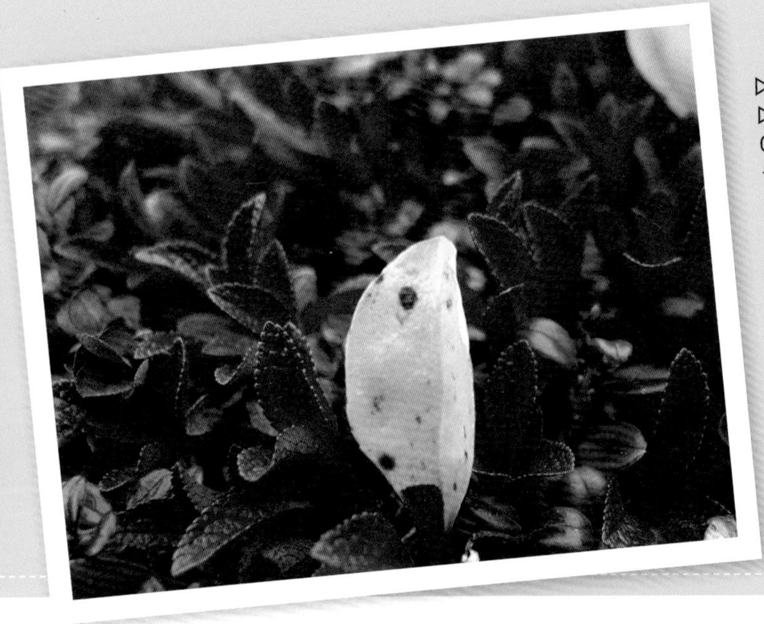

ᐅᑭᐊᒃᓵᒃᑯᑦ, ᐅᖅᐱᐅᑉ ᓱᐳᑎᓪᓗ ᐅᖃᐅᔭᙱᑦ ᖁᖅᓱᖅᑐᑦ ᑕᖅᓴᐅᑦᑎᐊᖅᑐᐊᓗᐃᑦ ᑲᓪᓚᖁᑎᐅᑉ ᐊᐅᐸᖅᑐᐃᑦ ᐅᖃᐅᔭᙱᓐᓂᑦ (ᐅᖃᐅᔭᙱᑦ ᑲᓪᓚᖁᑎᐅᑉ).

In autumn, the yellow leaves of uqpi suputillu stand out amongst red *kallaquti* (the leaves of bearberry).

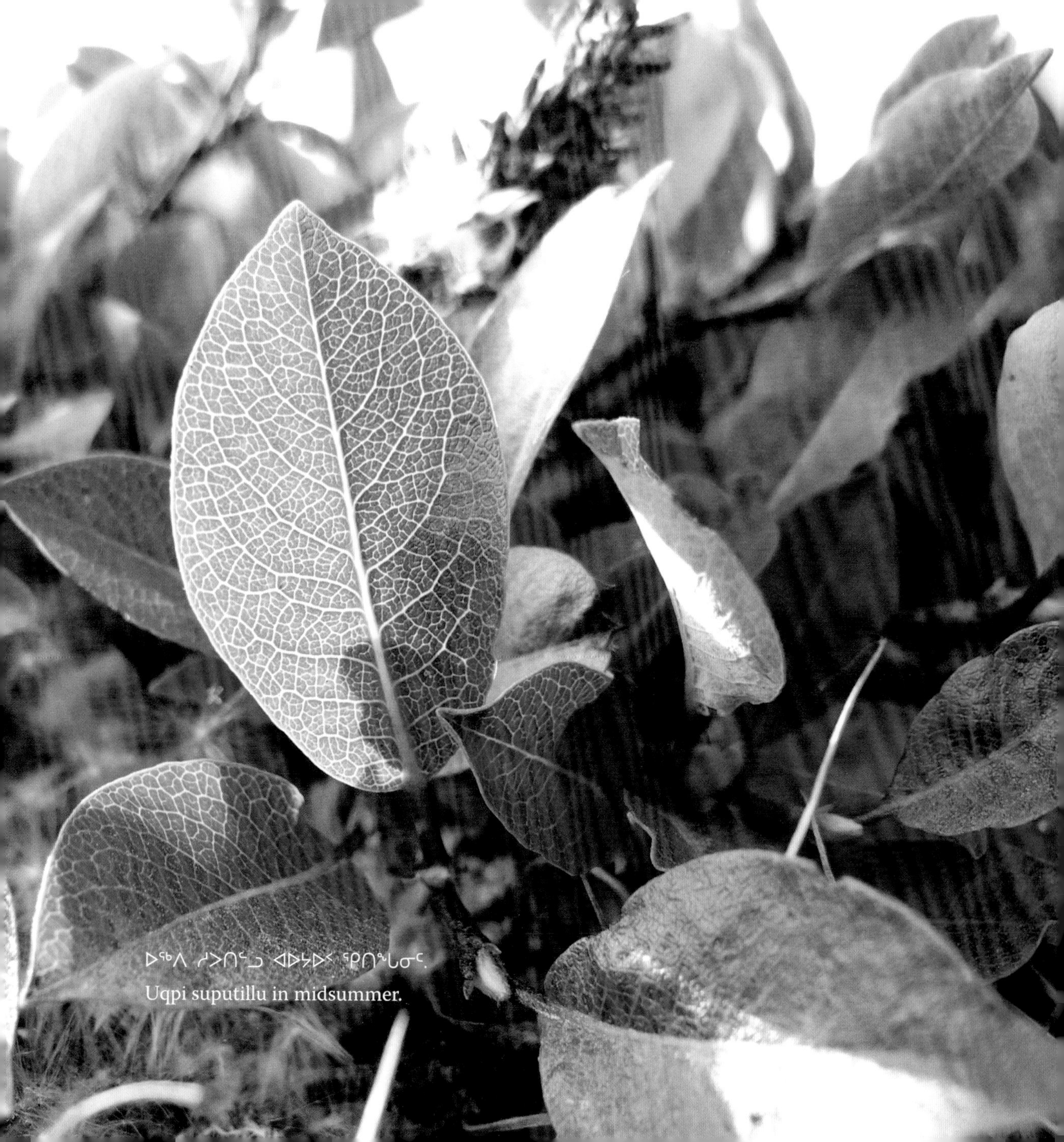

ᐅᖅᐱ ᓱᐳᑎᓪᓗ ᐊᐅᔭᐅᑉ ᕿᑎᖓᓂᑦ.

Uqpi suputillu in midsummer.

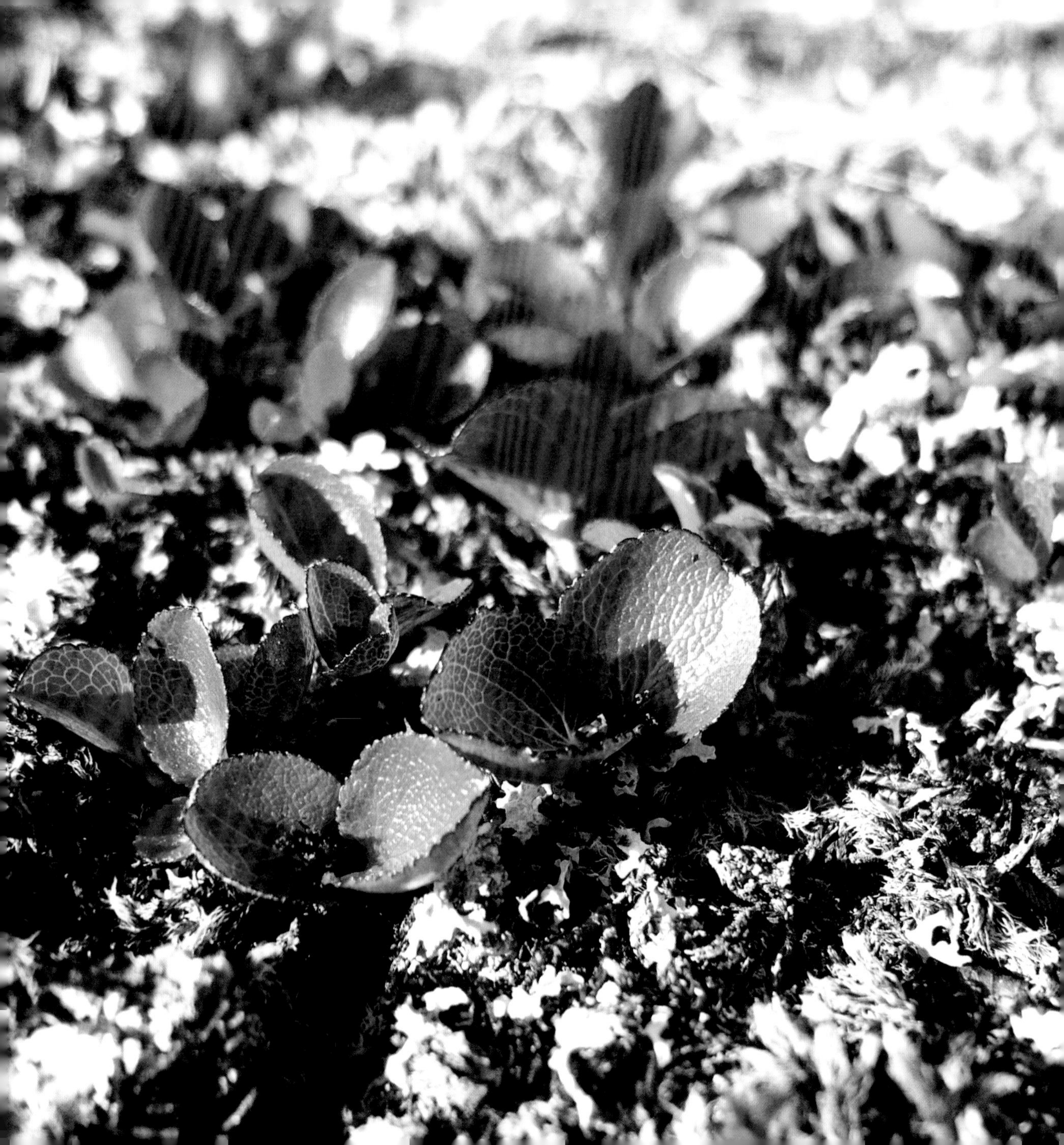

ᖁᐊᕋᐃᑦ

Quarait / Snow-Bed Willow

ᖁᐊᕋᐃᑦ ᒥᑭᑦᑐᑯᓘᑦ ᐅᒃᐱᒐᐅᓪᓗᓂᑦ ᐊᖏᓂᖓ 0.5ᒥᑦ 5 ᓯᐊᓐᑎᒦᑑᔪᓐᓇᖅᑐᖅ. ᐊᒻᒪᓗᐸᓗᒃᑐᑦ ᐅᖅᑲᐅᓯᖏᑦ 6ᒥᑦ 21 ᒥᓕᒦᑑᔪᓐᓇᖅᑐᑎᑦ ᑕᑭᓂᖏᑦ. ᑐᖑᑦᑐᓇᑦᑑᔪᑦ ᐅᖅᑲᐅᓯᖏᑕ ᑭᓪᓕᖏᑦ ᖃᑦᑎᒐᓛᑦᑐᑎᒃ. ᐱᕈᖅᓯᐊᖏᑦ ᐊᐅᐸᓪᓚᓇᑦᑐᑯᓗᐃᑦ ᐅᖅᑲᐅᓯᖏᓐᓃᖖᒑᖅᐸᑦᑐᑎᒃ, 5ᒥᑦ 11 ᒥᓕᒦᑐᒥᑦ ᑕᑭᓂᖅᑲᕈᓐᓇᖅᑐᑎᒃ. ᖁᐊᕋᐃᑦ ᐱᕈᒐᔪᑦᑐᑦ ᐊᐳᑎᓂᑦ ᐊᐅᓚᓵᖅᑐᕕᓂᕐᓂᑦ.

Quarait (snow-bed willow) are a very tiny willow that grow from 0.5 cm to 5 cm high. The nearly round leaves grow from 6 mm to 21 mm long. They are dark green with bumpy edges. The flowers are bright red catkins that grow up from the leaves, from 5 mm to 11 mm high. Quarait grow most commonly under late-snow beds.

ᖃᐅᕋᐃᑦ ᓂᖅᑭᑦᑎᐊᕙᒻᒪᕆᐅᔪᖅ ᒪᒪᖅᑐᑎᓪᓗ. ᐋᓚᓯ ᐃᖅᑲᐅᒪᔪᖅ ᐅᖅᑲᐅᓯᖏᓐᓂ ᓂᓃᓐᓇᖅᑲᑦᑕᓚᐅᕐᓂᖏᓐᓂᑦ ᓂᕕᐊᖅᓯᐊᖑᓪᓗᓂ. ᐊᒫᖏᑦ ᐅᖅᑲᐅᓯᖏᓪᓗ ᓂᖅᑭᑦᑎᐊᕙᐅᔪᑦ, ᑭᓯᐊᓂ ᑭᓪᓚᐸᖏᑦ ᐊᐅᐸᖅᑐᐃᑦ ᓂᖅᑭᐅᖏᑦᑐᑦ. ᐅᖅᑲᐅᓯᖏᑦ ᑕᐃᒫᑐᐃᓐᓇᖅ ᓂᕆᔭᒃᓴᐃᑦ ᐅᕝᕙᓘᓐᓃᑦ ᐃᓚᖓᐅᑎᓗᒋᑦ ᑲᑎᑕᐹᖑᑦ ᑐᖑᔪᖅᑕᖑᑦ ᐱᕈᖅᑐᕕᓂᕐᖑᑦ. ᐊᓗᓕᐊᓇᔭᒃᓴᐅᒻᒥᔪᑦ. ᐊᑯᑦᑎᓗᒋᓪᓕ ᐊᒡᒐᖕᖑᑦ ᐊᒃᓴᓕᓪᓗᒋᑦ ᐃᔅᓵᖅᑭᓇᓱᓐᓂᖏᓐᓂᑦ; ᐅᖅᓱᒧᑦ ᐃᓚᓕᐅᑎᓕᕐᒥᓗᒋᑦ.

Quarait are delicious and very nutritious. Aalasi recalls eating the leaves constantly when she was growing up. The rhizomes (underground stems) and leaves are both good to eat, but the catkins are not. The leaves can be eaten by themselves or with other greens. They can also be made into an alu. When using the leaves to make an alu, rub them between your palms first to release the juices; then, add them to the fat.

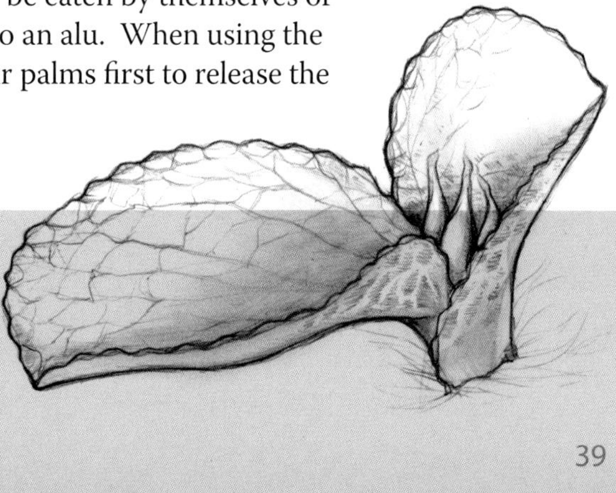

ᖁᐊᕋᐃᑦ ᑏᙳᐊᓕᐊᕆᔭᐅᖃᑦᑕᖕᒋᑦᑐᑦ. ᑭᓯᐊᓂᓕ ᐃᓚᓕᐅᑎᔭᕆᐊᐅᕗᑦ ᐃᖃᓗᖏᓂᓕᐅᖅᑕᓄᑦ.

Quarait are not used for tea. However, they can be added as a seasoning to the cooking water of boiled char.

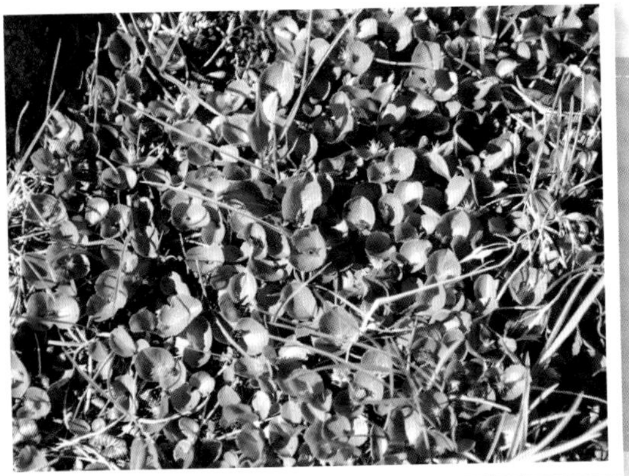

ᖁᐊᕋᐃᑦ ᒥᑭᓛᖑᕗᑦ ᓇᐹᖅᑐᓕᒫᓂᑦ ᓄᓇᕐᔪᐊᒥᑦ. ᐱᕈᒐᔪᓐᓂᖕᒥᑦ ᐊᐳᑎᖅᑯᑖᓯᓂᑦ ᖃᐅᔨᒪᔭᐅᔪᑦ, ᖄᓪᓗᓈᑎᑐᑦ ᐊᑎᖅᑲᖅᑐᑦ “ᐊᐳᒻᒥᑦ ᐃᓂᓖᑦ ᐱᕈᖅᓯᐊᑦ.”

Quarait are some of the tiniest trees in the world. They are known to grow where the snow remains longer than it does in surrounding areas, so this plant’s English name is “snow-bed willow.”

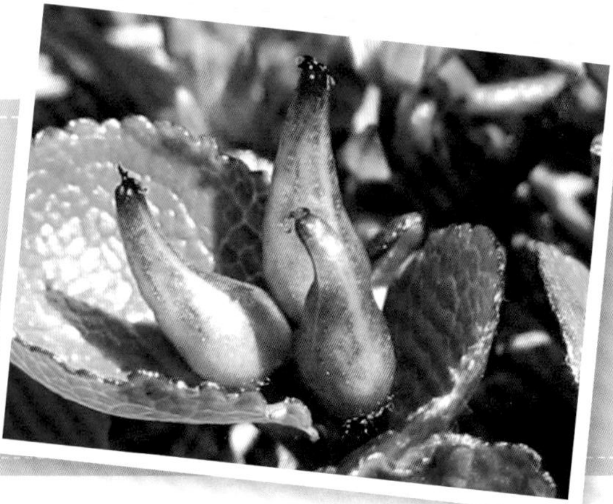

ᖁᐊᕋᐃᑦ ᒥᑭᑦᑐᕋᓛᑯᓗᐃᑦ ᐊᐅᐸᖅᑐᑦ ᐱᕈᖅᑕᑦᑕᖅᑐᑦ ᐅᖅᑲᐅᔭᓂᑦ.

Quarait have tiny red catkins that grow up from the leaves.

ᖁᐊᕋᐃᑦ ᐊᓗᒃ
Quarait Alu

- 1 ᐊᒡᒐ ᑕᑕᓪᓗᒍ ᖁᐊᕋᐃᑦ ᐅᖅᑲᐅᔭᖕᒋᓐᓂ
- 2 ᐊᓘᑎᑯᔅᓱᑦ ᓇᑦᑎᐅᑉ ᐊᐅᖕᒐ
- 1 ᐃᖕᒍᓯᖅ ᓇᑦᑎᐅᑉ ᐅᖅᓱᖕᒐ, ᑭᓱᑐᐃᓐᓇᐅᓪᓘᓐᓃᑦ ᐅᖅᓱᖕᒑᖕᒐᓂᑦ

- 1 handful of quarait leaves
- 2 tablespoons of seal blood
- 1 cup of seal fat or other fat

ᓯᕗᓪᓕᖅ, ᐅᖅᑲᐅᔭᖕᒋᑦ ᐊᒡᒐᓐᓂᑦ ᐊᒃᓴᓪᓗᑎᑦ ᐃᒃᓵᖅᑭᓕᕋᓱᓐᓂᖕᒋᓐᓂᑦ. ᐃᖕᒍᓚᖅᕕᒪᒍᑦ ᑲᑎᓪᓗᑎᑦ ᐅᖅᑲᐅᔭᑦ ᓇᑦᑎᐅᓪᓗ ᐊᐅᖕᒐ. ᐃᓚᓕᐅᑎᕙᓪᓕᐊᕋᔫᓪᓗᒍ ᓇᑦᑎᐅᑉ ᐅᖅᓱᖕᒐ, ᐊᓘᑎᕋᓛᒥᑦ ᐊᑐᖅᓗᑎᑦ, ᐊᑯᑎᐊᖅᓗᒍ. ᓂᕆᑐᐃᓐᓇᕋᒃᓴᐅᔪᑦ ᐃᓛᒃᑯᑦ ᐅᕝᕙᓘᓐᓃᑦ ᐆᔪᖅᑐᓕᕈᕕᑦ ᓂᕆᔭᒃᓴᐅᔪᓐᓇᖅᑐᖅ.

First, prepare the leaves by rubbing them between your palms until the juices are released from the leaves. Combine the leaves with the seal blood in a bowl. Slowly add the fat, spoonful by spoonful, combining well. Enjoy by itself or as a side dish with meat.

ᐋᓚᓯ ᒪᒪᑕᕐᑐᖅ ᖁᐊᕋᕐᓂᑦ ᔪᓚᐃ ᕿᑎᖕᒐᓂᑦ.

Aalasi enjoying quarait in mid-July.

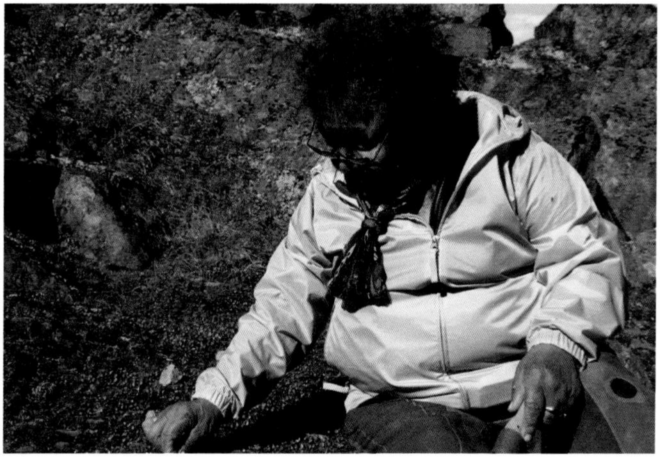

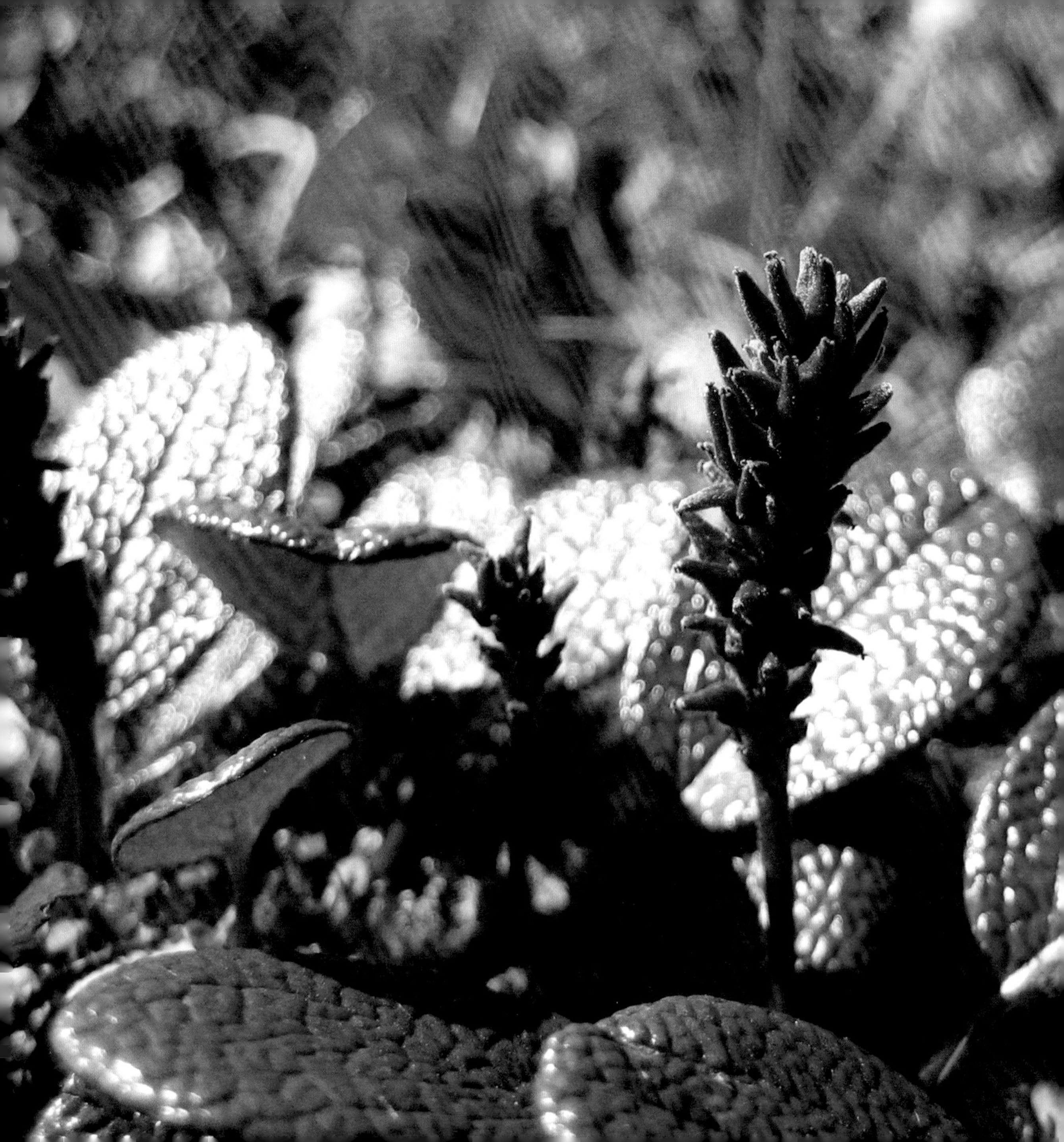

ᐊᓚᒃᓴᐅᔭᐃᑦ
Alaksaujait / Net-Vein Willow

ᐊᓚᒃᓴᐅᔭᐃᑦ ᑐᖑᔪᖅᑕᕈᔪᑯᓗᒻᒥᑦ ᐊᒥᐊᖅᑲᖅᑐᑦ ᐊᒻᒪᓗᕿᓵᕈᔫᓪᓗᑎᒃ. ᐅᖅᑲᐅᓯᖏᑦ ᖅᑭᓪᓕᕈᔭᒃᑐᑎᒃ ᑕᖅᑲᙱᐊᓕᐊᔫᓪᓗᑎᒃ ᓄᓗᐊᑎᑐᑦ ᐋᖅᑭᒃᓱᖅᓯᒪᔭᓂᒃ. ᐱᕈᖅᑲᑦᑕᖅᑐᑦ ᓄᓇᐅᑉ ᖅᑳᖓᒍᑦ. ᐊᒥᐊᖏᑦ ᖅᑯᖅᓱᖅᑑᖅᑲᑦᑕᖅᑐᑦ ᑲᔪᕈᔫᓪᓗᑎᑦ ᐅᕝᕙᓘᓐᓃᑦ ᐊᐅᐸᖅᑑᓪᓗᑎᑦ ᑲᔪᕈᔫᓂᖅᑲᖅᑐᑎᒃ. ᐊᓚᒃᓴᐅᔭᐃᑦ ᑭᓪᓚᐸᓖᑦ ᐊᐅᐸᓪᓚᕆᑦᑐᓂᑦ ᐅᖅᑲᐅᓯᖏᓐᓂᙵᖅᑲᑦᑕᖅᑐᑎᒃ, 4 ᓯᐊᓐᑎᒦᑐᒥᑦ ᐊᖏᓂᖅᓴᐅᓕᕈᓐᓇᖅᑎᑦ.

Alaksaujait (net-vein willow) are easily recognizable by their shiny, bright green leaves, marked deeply with veins in a net-like pattern. The leaves are almost round, reaching a gentle point at the tip. The branches grow along the ground. They are smooth and can be yellow brown or red brown. Alaksaujait have small, dark red catkins that grow up slightly from the leaves (usually no more than 4 cm).

ᑏᙳᐊᑐᐃᓐᓇᐅᓗᐊᖅᑲᑦᑕᖅᑐᑦ ᐊᓚᒃᓴᐅᔭᐃᑦ. ᐅᖅᑲᐅᓯᖏᑦ, ᓇᑲᖏᑦ ᐊᐃᕋᖏᑦᓗ ᓄᐊᑕᐅᒍᓐᓇᖅᑐᑦ ᐊᐅᔭᐅᑉ ᖅᑭᑎᐊᓂᑦ ᓄᙳᐊᓄᑦ. ᐃᓕᒃᑯᐊᕆᔭᐅᖅᑲᑦᑕᕈᓐᓇᖅᒥᔪᑦ ᐅᑭᐅᓕᒫᖅᑯᑦ. ᐋᓚᓯ ᐃᖅᑲᐅᒪᔪᖅ ᐊᖑᓇᓱᑦᑏᑦ ᑕᖅᑯᐊᖅᑲᑦᑕᓚᐅᖅᓂᖏᓐᓂᑦ ᐊᓚᒃᓴᐅᔭᓂᑦ ᐊᐅᓪᓚᖅᓯᒪᓂᖏᓐᓂᑦ ᐱᔭᐅᖅᑲᑦᑕᖅᓂᐊᖅᑐᓂᒃ. ᐅᖅᑲᐅᓯᖏᑦ ᐆᖅᑕᐅᓯᒪᖅᑲᑦᑕᖅᑐᕕᓃᑦ ᖅᑭᓯᔭᓂᑦ ᐆᑲᒻᒫᓗᖕᓄᑦ.

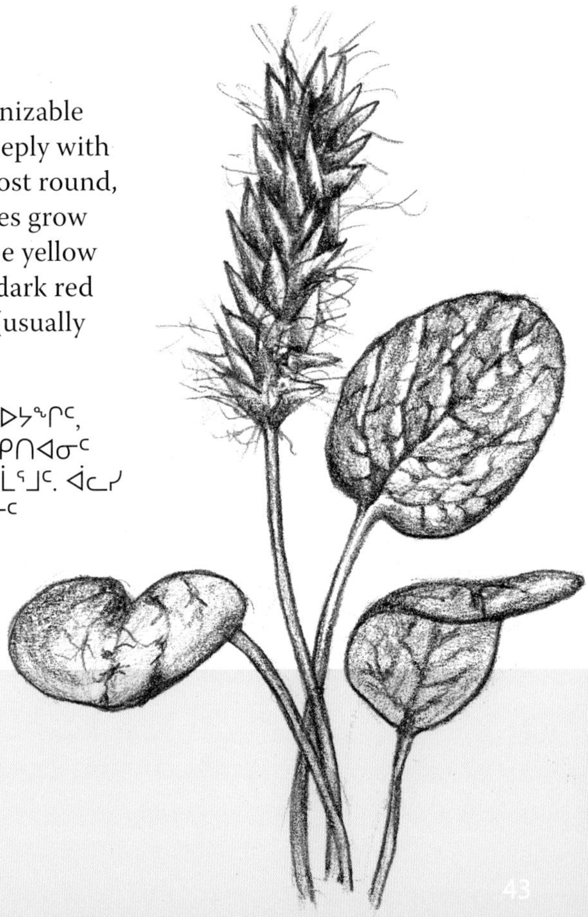

The primary use of alaksaujait is to make tea. The leaves, stems, and roots can be gathered and used from mid- to late summer. They can also be stored for later use during the winter. Aalasi recalls that hunters would take alaksaujait with them on their trips to drink while they were away. They would store the leaves in sealskin purses.

ᐊᓚᒃᓴᐅᔭᐃᑦ ᑏᓐᖑᐊᖕᖑᓪᓗᑎᑦ ᓴᓐᖏᔪᒻᒪᓃᑦ ᑎᒥᒧᓪᓗ ᐊᑑᑎᖃᑦᑎᐊᖅᑐᑎᒃ ᐊᒻᒪ ᐊᑲᐅᓯᓴᐅᑎᐅᑦᑎᐊᕆᓪᓗᑎᒃ ᖃᓄᐃᓐᓇᖅ ᐋᓐᓂᐊᔪᓄᑦ ᓈᖅᓱᓐᓇᖅᑐᓄᑦ ᐱᓗᐊᖅᑐᓂ. ᑎᒥᒥᑦ ᐊᐅᒪᔾᔭᑦᑎᒃᑎᓲᖑᔪᑦ, ᑎᒥᒧᑦ ᑕᒪᓐᓇ ᐊᑲᐅᓯᓴᐅᑎᐅᓪᓗᓂ. ᓴᓐᖏᓗᐊᒧᑦ ᐋᒪᒪᑦᑎᑦᑎᔪᖅ ᑏᑐᕐᓂᕈᓂ ᐋᒪᒪᑦᑎᑕᖓ ᓄᑕᖅ ᐊᑦᑐᖅᑕᐅᒐᔭᖅᑐᖅ.

Alaksaujait tea is a strong tea that can help with almost all illnesses, especially illnesses that involve an upset stomach. The tea creates body heat and causes a person to sweat, which is good for their health. This tea is powerful enough that its effects may be felt by a breastfeeding baby whose mother has drunk the tea.

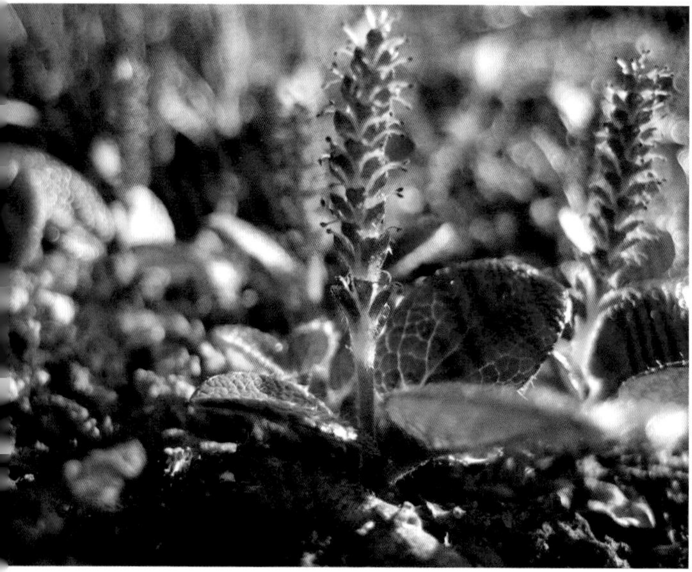

ᑏᓐᖑᐊᓕᐅᕐᓂᐊᕐᓗᓂᓕ ᐊᓚᒃᓴᐅᔭᓂᑦ, ᓄᐊᑦᑎᓚᐅᕐᓗᑎᑦ ᐊᒡᒐᐃᑦ ᑕᑕᓗᐊᕐᓗᒍ ᐅᖅᑲᐅᔭᓂᑦ, ᓇᑲᖕᖏᓐᓂᑦ ᐊᐃᖁᖕᖏᓐᓂᓪᓗ (ᑭᓪᓚᐸᖕᖏᑦ ᐱᖅᑯᓯᐅᑎᖕᖏᓪᓗᒋᑦ). ᐃᒪᖅ ᑎᖅᑎᑎᓪᓗᒍ ᐃᓱᖅᓯᕈᔪᒐᓱᓐᓂᖕᒐᓂ—ᐅᔾᔨᓇᒐᔭᖅᑕᒃᓴᓇᕚᑦ ᑖᓐᓇ ᑏᓐᖑᐊᖕᖑᓗᒍ ᐊᔾᔨᐅᑦᑎᐊᖕᖏᑦᑐᑯᓘᒻᒪᑦ.

ᐊᓚᒃᓴᐅᔭᐃᑦ ᐅᓐᓄᓕᖅᑎᓪᓗᒍ ᐃᖃᓗᐃᑦ ᓴᓂᐊᓂᑦ ᐊᐅᔭᐅᑉ ᖁᑎᖕᒐᓂᑦ.

Alaksaujait at dusk in midsummer near Iqaluit.

To make tea from alaksaujait, collect a generous handful of leaves, stems, and roots (but not catkins). Boil them until the water has thickened slightly—you will probably notice the unique consistency of tea made from this plant.

ᐊᐃᕋᖕᒋᑦᑕᐅᑉ ᑖᒃᓯᒪᑦ ᐱᕈᖅᑰᑉ ᓂᕿᑦᑎᐊᕙᐅᔪᑦ. ᒪᒪᖅᑐᒃᑰᑦᑐᑎᑦ ᑕᐃᒫᑐᐃᓐᓇ ᓂᕆᒋᐊᖕᖓ.

The leaves and roots of this plant are also nutritious. They are enjoyable to eat fresh and raw.

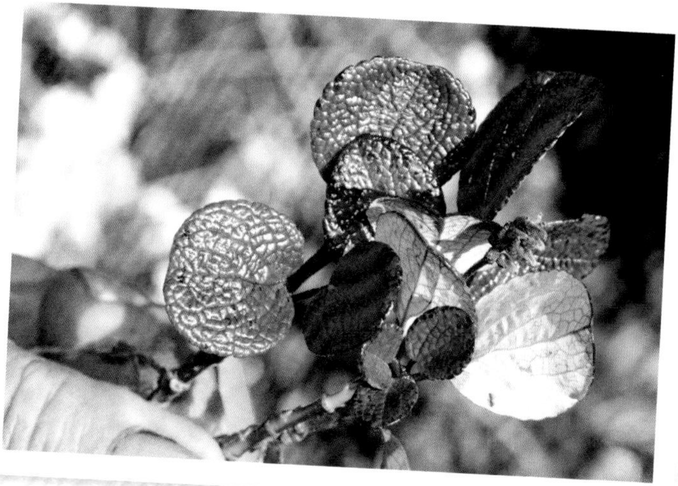

ᐊᓚᒃᓴᐅᔭᐃᑦ ᐱᑐᕐᑐᒍ ᑎᒥᒥᑦ ᐊᐅᒪᔾᔭᑦᑎᒃᑎᓲᖕᒍᔪᑦ, ᐋᓐᓂᐊᒥᑦ ᑕᐃᒪ ᐊᓂᐊᑦᑎᔪᖅ, ᐱᓗᐊᖅᑐᒥᒃ ᓈᕐᑐᑦᑐᓂ.

Tea from alaksaujait creates body heat and causes a person to sweat out illnesses, especially those related to the stomach.

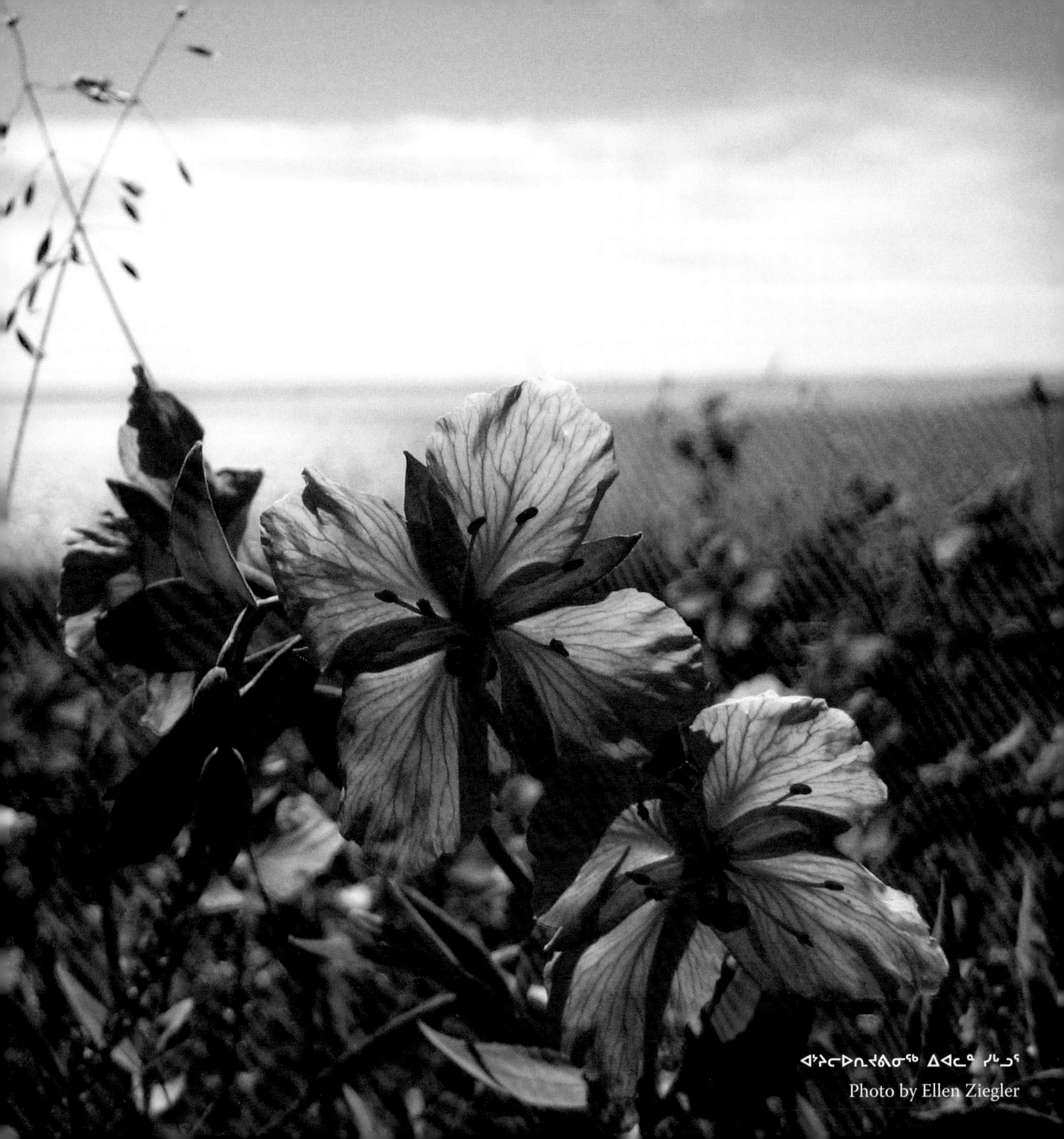

ᐊᔾᔨᓕᐅᕆᔪᕕᓂᖅ ᐃᐊᓚᓐ ᓯᒡᓗᕐ
Photo by Ellen Ziegler

ᐸᐅᓐᓇᐃᑦ
Paunnait / Dwarf Fireweed

ᐸᐅᓐᓇᐃᑦ ᐅᑭᐅᖅᑕᖅᑐᒥᑦ ᓇᓂᔭᐅᓖᖕᔪᕗᑦ. ᐱᕈᒐᕙᒃᑐᑦ ᓯᐅᕋᕐᒥᑦ ᓲᕐᕋᒃᑕᐅᓯᒪᕙᓂᑦ, ᐅᔾᔨᕆᓚᒐᔭᖅᑕᒃᓴᕆᓚᔭᑎᑦ ᓄᓇᓕᖕᓂᑦ ᐊᖅᑯᑎᐅᑉ ᑭᒡᓕᖕᒐᓂ. ᓄᓇᓖᑦᓕ ᓯᓚᑖᓂᑦ ᖃᖅᑲᔮᓃᓰᑦ, ᓯᐅᕋᔮᒥᓪᓘᓐᓃᑦ ᓯᔾᔭᒥ. ᐱᕈᓕᖓᖅᑎᓪᓗᒍ ᐅᐱᕐᖔᒃᑯᑦ ᐸᐅᓐᓇᑦ ᐊᐅᐸᓪᓚᓴᑦᑐᑰᖅᑲᑦᑕᖅᑐᑦ. ᑕᕐᕋᓕ ᑐᖑᔭᖅᑕᕈᕌᖕᒐᑕ, ᐱᕈᖅᓯᐊᖕᒥᑦ ᐱᕈᓇᖅᑲᑦᑕᖅᑐᑦ. ᑖᒃᑯᐊᓕ ᓇᒥᑐᐃᓐᓇ ᔭᓚᐃ ᕿᑎᖅᐸᓯᖕᒐᓂ ᐱᕈᓇᑦᑎᐊᖅᑲᑦᑕᖅᑐᑦ ᐋᒡᒌᓯᐅᓕᕋᖕᒐ ᑭᓯᐊᓂᑦ ᑐᖁᓕᕐᑦᑐᑎᒃ.

Paunnait (dwarf fireweed) are found across the Arctic. This plant tends to grow where the soil has been disturbed, so you might notice it near roads and waterways around your community. Out on the land, this plant grows on exposed hillsides and on gravelly shores. When they first begin to grow in the spring, the stalks and leaves of paunnait are dark red. Then they turn green and their flowers begin to open. In most regions, the flowers open in mid-July and remain until late August.

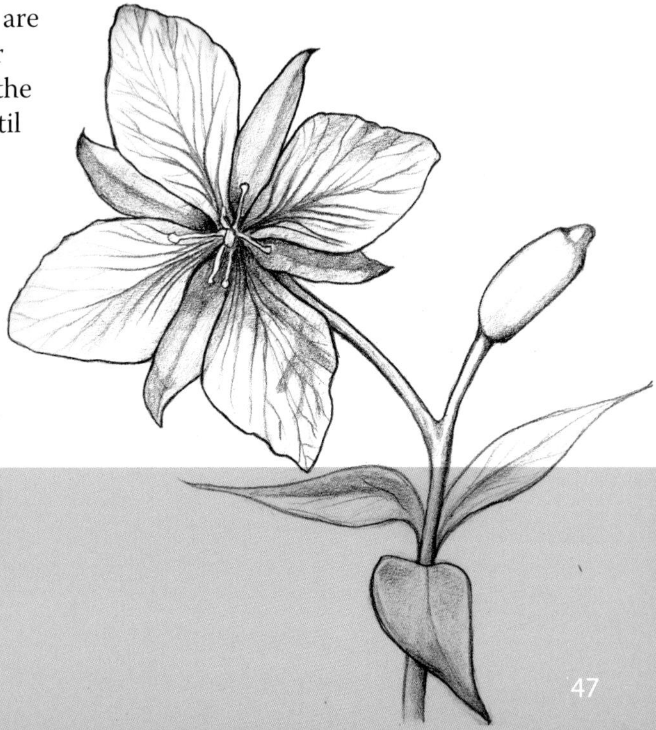

ᐸᐅᓐᓇᑦ 5 ᓯᐊᓐᑎᒦᑐᓂᑦ 30ᓯᐊᓐᑎᒦᑐᓄᑦ ᐊᖏᓂᑖᕈᓐᓇᖅᑐᑦ. ᐸᐅᓐᓇᐃᑦ ᐅᖅᑲᐅᔭᖏᑦ ᑐᖑᔭᖅᑕᐅᓪᓗᑎᒃ ᑭᓪᓕᖏᑦ ᓂᕈᒥᑦᑑᓪᓗᑎᒃ. ᐃᓛᓐᓂᒃᑯᑦ ᑕᑭᔪᑯᑖᑯᓘᖅᑲᑦᑕᖅᑐᑦ ᐃᓛᓐᓂᒃᑯᓪᓗ ᓇᐃᑦᑑᓪᓗᑎᒃ ᓯᓕᑦᑐᑲᓪᓚᐅᓪᓗᑎᓪᓗ.

ᐱᕈᖅᓯᐊᖑᓂᖏᑦ ᐊᖏᔫᓪᓗᑎᑦ (2-5 ᓯᐊᓐᑎᒦᑐᒦᑐᑎᒃ ᑕᑭᓂᖏᑦ) ᐊᐅᐸᕈᔪᒃᑑᖅᑲᑦᑕᖅᑐᑦ, ᐊᐅᐸᓪᓚᕆᑦᑐᑎᓪᓗ. ᑎᓴᒪᐅᑕᖕᒐᔪᓂᑦ ᐱᕈᖅᑐᖅᑲᖅᐸᑦᑐᑎᒃ ᐊᒻᒪᓗ ᐊᑦᑕᑎᖏᑦ ᑕᖅᓴᐅᓂᖅᓴᐅᓪᓗᑎᑦ ᐊᐅᐸᕈᔪᒃᑑᓪᓗᑎᑦ. ᐸᐅᓐᓇᐃᑦ ᐊᖏᔫᒻᒪᑕ ᑕᑯᔭᕐᓂᖅᑐᑯᓗᐃᑦ.

Paunnait grow between 5 cm and 30 cm tall. The leaves are bluish green and have smooth edges. They can be long and narrow, and they can also be shorter and oval shaped. The flowers are large (2 cm to 5 cm across) and they are bright pink or purple. The flowers have four wide petals and four darker pink sepals (special leaves that enclose the flower bud). Because the flowers are so large and bright, paunnait are easy to spot.

ᐸᐅᓐᓇᐃᑦ ᐊᑑᑎᓪᓚᒪᓈᑦ. ᓂᕿᑦᑎᐊᕙᐅᓪᓗᑎᒃ ᑎᒥᒧᓪᓗ ᐱᐅᓪᓗᑎᒃ.

Paunnait have many uses. They are an all-purpose source of nutrition and are good for overall health.

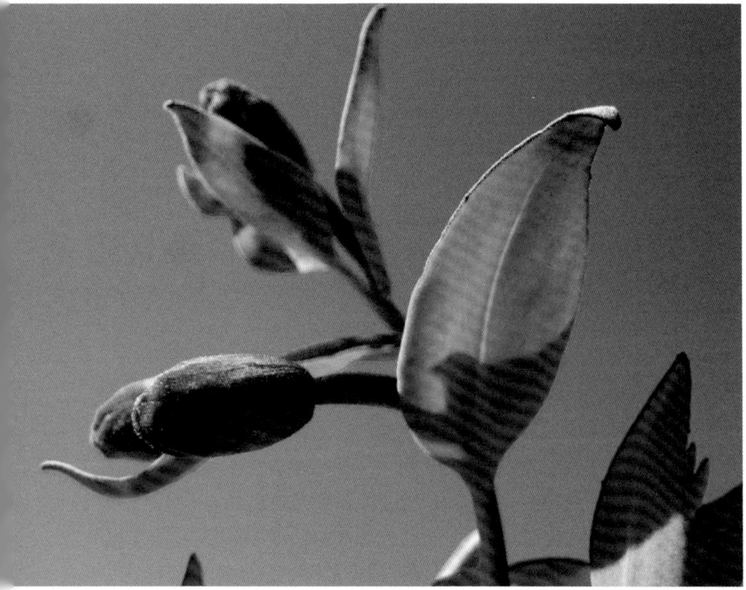

ᑐᖑᔪᖅᑕᐅᓂᖏᑦ ᓂᕆᔭᐅᔪᓐᓇᖅᑐᑦ ᑕᐃᒫᑐᐃᓐᓇᖅ ᐊᓘᓗᒍᓘᓐᓃᑦ ᐅᖅᓱᒥᒃ ᐊᒻᒪᓗ ᐊᐅᒻᒥᑦ ᐃᓚᓯᒪᓗᒍ.

The green parts of the plant can be eaten plain and they can also be mixed with fats and blood to make nutritious side dishes.

ᐸᐅᓐᓇᐃᑦ ᐱᕈᖅᓯᐊᒃᓴᖅᑲᓚᓲᑦ ᔪᓚᐃ ᐱᒋᐊᕐᓂᖓᓂ.

The buds of paunnait in early July.

ᐸᐅᓐᓇᐃᑦ ᐊᒫᖏᑦ ᑕᐃᒫᑐᐃᓐᓇᖅ ᓂᕆᔭᒃᓴᐃᑦ. ᓄᑕᕋᕐᓅᖅᑕᐅᔪᓐᓇᕐᒥᔪᑦ ᐊᒫᒪᕋᐅᔭᕆᔭᐅᑎᑦᓗᒋᑦ. ᓄᑕᕋᕐᓘᖅᑕᐅᓂᐊᕈᓂ ᐊᒫᖅ ᑕᑭᔫᒋᐊᕐᓗᒍ ᑐᐱᔾᔪᑕᐅᔪᓐᓇᖅᑎᒋᐊᖏᑦᓗᒍ. ᓇᐃᑦᓚᓗᐊᓚᕈᓂᓚ ᑭᒻᒪᓚᓂᐅᓗᐊᓚᕈᓂᓘᓐᓃᑦ ᓄᑕᖅ ᐋᕐᑯᔭᖅ. ᐊᒫᖅ ᑭᒍᓯᓴᔭᒥᒃ ᐃᑲᔪᕐᓇᖅᑐᖅ ᐊᒻᒪᓗ ᓂᖅᑭᑦᑎᐊᕙᐅᑦᓗᓂ.

The rhizomes of paunnait can be eaten just as they are. They can also be given to babies as pacifiers. If a rhizome is given to a baby, it should be fairly long so that it is not easy to swallow. Also, it should be taken away before it has been chewed down too much. The rhizomes help with teething and they also provide nutrients.

ᐸᐅᓐᓇᐃᑦ ᑏᖖᒍᐊᑦᑎᐊᕚᓘᒐᑦ, ᑎᒥᑦᑎᐊᕆᓐᓇᖅᑐᑎᒃ. ᑎᒥᒧᑦ ᐊᑑᑎᖅᑲᑦᑎᐊᕐᓂᖓᓄᑦ ᐸᐅᓐᓇ ᑎᖑᓗᒍᑦ ᓄᑕᕋᕐᒧᑦ ᐊᑐᖅᑕᐅᔪᓐᓇᖅᑐᖅ ᐃᒻᒧᒋᔭᐅᖓᕐᓗᓂ ᐃᒻᒧᖅᑲᖏᑦᑐᒧ. ᐃᓄᐃᑦ ᐃᓚᖏᑦ ᐅᓪᓗᑕᒫᖅ ᑏᑐᖅᑲᑦᑕᖅᑐᑦ ᐸᐅᓐᓇᕐᓂᑦ ᑎᒥᑦᑎᐊᕆᒍᒪᓪᓗᑎᑦ. ᐸᐅᓐᓇᐃᑦ ᑏᖖᒍᐊᓕᐅᕐᓂᐊᕈᕕᑦ ᓄᐊᑦᑎᖅᑳᕆᐊᕐᑲᖅᐳᑎ. ᐅᐊᓯᕐᓗᒋᑦ ᓴᓃᔭᑦᑎᐊᕐᓗᒋᑦ, ᐱᕈᖅᓯᐊᖏᑦ ᐲᔭᕐᓗᒋᑦ ᐊᒫᖏᓪᓗ. ᐸᐅᓐᓇᐃᑦ ᐅᖃᐅᔭᐅᓂᖏᑦ ᑎᖅᑎᑎᓪᓗᒋᑦ ᐃᖁᕐᓂᖓ ᓈᒻᒪᒋᓕᕋᓱᓐᓂᕐᓂᑦ. ᒪᒪᑕᓐᓂᐊᖅᐳᑎᕐ!

Paunnait can be boiled into a delicious tea that is very good for overall health. A very strong paunnait tea can even replace milk or

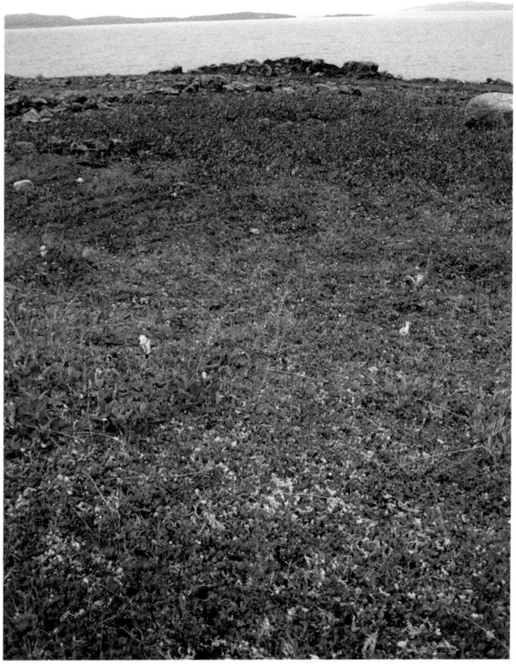

ᐸᐅᓐᓇᐃᑦ ᓇᓗᓇᖏᑦᑎᐊᖅᑐᑦ
ᐊᖏᔫᒻᒪᑕ ᐊᒥᐊᖏᑦᓗ ᑕᖅᓴᐅᑦᓗᑎᑦ.

Paunnait are easily recognizable by their large size and bright colour.

formula for babies because it is so high in nutrients. Some people drink this tea every day for good health. To make delicious paunnait tea, gather several of the plants. Rinse them to remove any dust, remove any flowers or rhizomes, and then boil all the leaves until the desired strength of tea is reached. Enjoy!

ᐊᐅᓭᓪᓛᖅ ᐸᐅᓐᓇᐃᑦ ᓄᐊᒐᒃᓴᐅᕗᑦ ᑭᓯᐊᓂᑦ ᐱᐅᓂᖅᐹᖑᕗᑦ ᓄᐊᑎᐊᖓ ᐅᐱᕐᖔ ᓄᙳᐸᓗᐊᒍᑦ ᐱᑐᖅᓯᐊᖏᑦ ᑲᑕᒃᓯᒪᓂᖅᑎᑦᓗᒋᑦ ᐅᖅᑲᐅᓭᖏᑦ ᑐᖑᔪᖅᑕᐅᑎᑦᓗᒋᑦ ᓯᓂ. ᑕᕝᕙ ᑕᐃᒪᐃᑎᑦᓗᒋᑦ ᐸᐅᓐᓇᐃᑦ ᐊᑲᐅᓯᓴᐅᑎᖃᕐᓂᖅᐹᖑᕗᑦ ᐊᒻᒪᓗ ᒪᒪᖅᓯᑦᑎᐊᖅᓯᒪᑦᓗᑎᑦ. ᓄᐊᑕᐅᓚᐅᖅᑎᑦᓗᒋᑦ ᓴᓂᕐᕙᒐᒃᓴᐅᕗᑦ ᐅᑭᐅᓪᓛᕐᒧᑦ.

Although you can collect paunnait to make tea all summer, the best time to collect it is in the very late summer when the flowers are gone but the leaves are still green. At this time, it has the most flavour and medicinal strength. Once collected, the leaves can be saved and used for tea all winter.

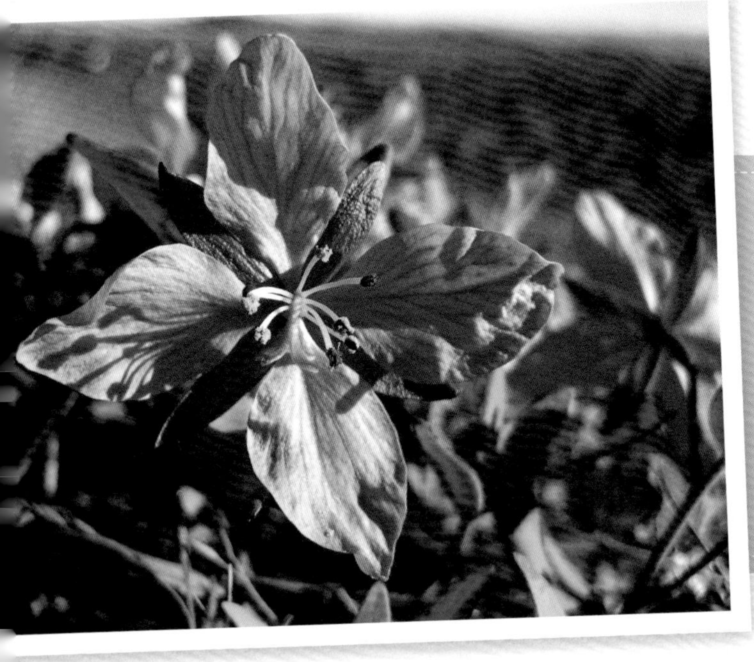

ᐊᑲᐅᓯᓴᐅᑕᐅᓂᐊᖅᑎᓪᓗᒋᓪᓚ, ᐸᐅᓈᐃᑦ ᑎᖅᑎᑦᑐᒦᑯᑖᑦᑎᓪᓗᒋᑦ ᐃᒪᖓ ᐃᓱᓪᓚᓇᓕᖅᑎᓪᓗᒍ. ᑖᓐᓇ ᐊᑲᐅᓯᕚᓪᓕᖅᑎᑦᑎᔾᔪᓇᖅᑐᖅ ᓈᕐᓗᑦᑐᓂᒃ ᐊᔾᔨᒌᖏᑦᑐᓂᒃ. ᑏᖖᒍᐊᖑᓪᓗᑎ ᓈᕐᓗᑦᑐᓄᑦ ᐊᓇᕈᓇᐃᓕᓯᒪᔪᓄᑦ ᐊᑐᖅᑕᐅᒐᔪᑦᑐᖅ. ᐅᖃᐅᔾᔭᖏᑦ ᐸᐅᓇᐅᑉ ᓂᕆᑐᐃᓐᓇᕐᓗᒋᑦ ᓈᖖᒍᔪᒧᑦ ᐊᑲᐅᓱᔾᔪᑕᐅᔾᔪᓇᕐᒥᔪᑦ.

For medicinal uses, boil the leaves until the mixture is very dark. This will produce a tea that can help with many ailments, especially those related to the stomach. This tea is commonly known to help with constipation. Simply eating a handful of the leaves will also help an upset stomach.

ᐸᐅᓈᐃᑦ ᖃᐅᔨᒪᔭᐅᕆᕙᑦ ᓂᐊᖅᑯᖖᒍᔪᓄᑦ ᐊᑐᖅᑕᐅᔾᔪᓇᕐᓂᖏᑦ. ᓂᐊᕐᑯᖅᓯᐅᑕᐅᓂᐊᖅᑎᓪᓗᒍᓚ ᐸᐅᓇᖅ ᑎᖅᑎᑎᓪᓗᒍ ᐃᓱᓪᓚᓇᓕᕋᓱᓐᓂᖓᓂ, ᕿᕐᓂᖅᑑᓗᓂᓗ. ᑎᓴᐃᖅᑎᓚᐅᕐᓗᒍ, ᐆᓇᕋᓗᐊᕐᓗᓂ (ᐆᓇᓗᐊᖖᒋᓱᖕᒐᖅᐸ ᐊᑐᕐᓂᐊᖅᑐᒧᑦ), ᖃᓪᓗᓈᖅᑕᖅ ᒪᓯᒃᑎᕐᓗᒍ, ᑕᒪᓐᓇ ᖃᓪᓗᓈᖅᑕᖅ ᐃᓅᑉ ᓂᐊᕐᑯᖓᓄᑦ ᕿᓚᓪᓗᒍ.
ᐊᑲᐅᓯᓴᐅᑎᖓ ᑏᒦᑦᑑᑉ ᐅᕙᓂᒃᑯᑦ ᑎᒥᔫᖅᐸᓪᓚᐊᓂᐊᖅᑐᖅ. ᐆᓇᕐᓂᖓ ᑏ ᐃᓄᒻᒥᑦ ᐅᖅᑰᑎᑦᑎᓗᓂ ᐋᓂᐊᒥᑦ ᐊᓂᐊᑎᑦᑎᔾᔪᓇᖅᑐᖅ ᐊᐅᒃᑲᕐᓂᒃᑯᑦ.

ᐸᐅᓈᐃᑦ ᐱᕈᒡᒍᔪᑦ ᓯᐅᕋᕐᒥᑦ ᓱᕐᕋᑦᑕᐅᓯᒪᔪᓂᑦ, ᓲᕐᓗ ᐊᖅᑯᑎᑯᑖᑦ ᑭᓪᓕᖕᒋᓐᓂᒃ, ᐃᓪᓗᓕᐅᕐᕕᐅᔪᐃᑦ ᓴᓂᐊᓂᑦ, ᐊᓄᕖᒃᑲᕐᓂᓗ ᓄᓇᔾᔭᒥᑦ. ᐊᔾᔨᓕᐅᕆᔪᕕᓂᖅ ᓃᑦ ᑯᓇᔅᑕᕗᖅ.

Paunnait grow in places where the soil has been disturbed, such as along roadsides, near construction sites, and on windswept ridges of the tundra.

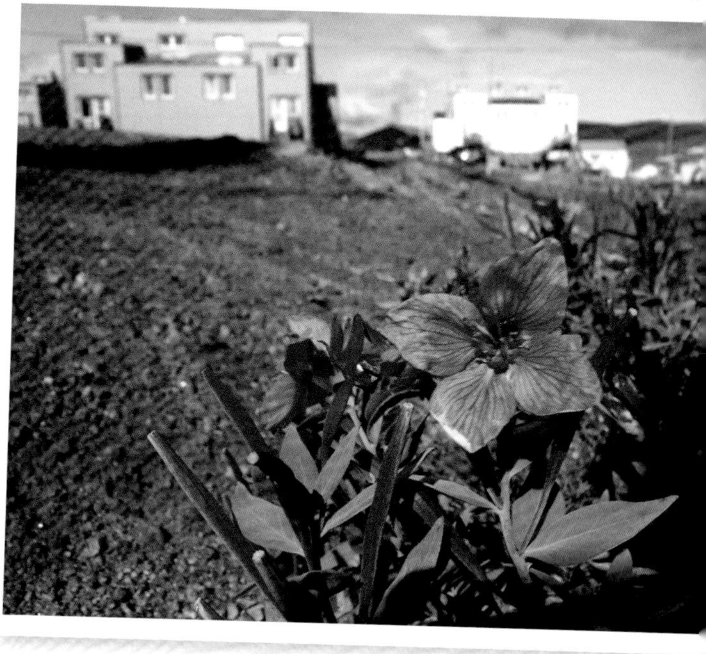

Paunnait are known to help with very bad headaches. To use paunnait for a headache, boil a very dark and thick tea. When the tea is still hot (as hot as the person can tolerate), soak a cloth in the tea. Wrap the soaked cloth around the person's head. The nutrients in the tea will be absorbed through the skin. The sweating caused by the warmth of the tea will also help.

ᐸᐅᓐᓇᐃᑦ ᐅᖅᑲᐅᔭᖕᒋᑦ ᒪᑦᑐᑎᐅᖅᑲᑦᑕᕐᒥᔪᑦ ᑭᓚᖅᓯᒪᔪᒧᑦ, ᑭᑦᑐᓇᐊᖅᑕᐅᓯᒪᔪᒧᑦ ᐊᒻᒪᓗ ᐊᓯᖕᒋᓐᓄᑦ ᐅᕙᓂᒻᒧᑦ ᑐᕌᖕᒐᔪᑦ ᐊᑯᐅᖖᒋᓚᐅᕈᑎᑦ. ᐅᐊᓴᓚᐅᖅᑎᑦᑐᒋᑦ ᐅᖅᑲᐅᔭᖕᒋᑦ ᑭᓚᖅᒧᑦ ᐃᓚᑐᒍ. ᓄᐊᕋᑖᖅᓯᒪᔪᑦ ᐅᖅᑲᐅᔭᐃᑦ ᑕᐃᒫᒃ ᐊᑐᕋᒃᓴᐅᔪᑦ, ᑭᓯᐊᓂ ᓄᐊᓯᒪᔪᑦ ᐅᑭᐅᓚᒫᖅᒧᑦ ᐊᑐᐃᓐᓇᕆᔭᒃᓴᐅᒋᕗᑦ.

The leaves can also be used as small bandages to heal cuts, bug bites, or other skin irritations. After rinsing a leaf, place it on the cut or irritation. Fresh leaves can be used this way, but you can also save the leaves and use them as small bandages in the winter.

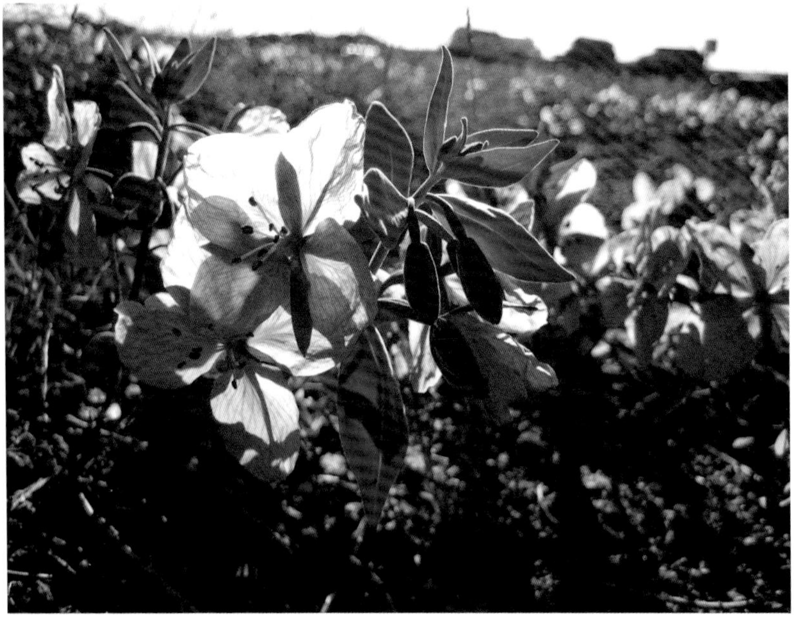

ᐸᐅᓐᓇᐃᑦ ᐃᓗᓚᐅᖕᒐᔪᒥᒃ, ᔪᓚᐃ ᕿᑎᖕᒐᓂ ᐃᖅᑲᓗᖕᓂᑦ.

Paunnait along a ditch, mid-July in Iqaluit.

ᐸᐅᓐᓇᐃᑦ ᐊᑯᓪᓗᒋᑦ
Paunnait Alu

ᐊᑰᑎᕐᑲᑦᑎᐊᖅᑐᖅ ᓂᕿᑦᑎᐊᕙᐅᓪᓗᓂᓗ, ᓂᕆᔭᒃᓴᐅᒐᑦ ᐆᔪᖅᑐᕐᓗᓂ ᑐᒃᑐᕚᓂᕐᒥᓘᓐᓃᑦ.

A nutritious side dish that can be served with caribou or other meat.

- 5 ᐸᐅᓐᓇᐃᑦ ᐅᕐᑲᐅᔭᖕᒋᑦ
- 2 ᐊᓘᑎᑯᔅᓯᒃ ᓇᑦᑎᐅᑉ ᐊᐅᖓ
- 1 ᐃᕐᖑᓯᖅ ᓇᑦᑎᐅᑉ ᐅᖅᓯᖓ

- Leaves of 5 paunnait
- 2 tablespoons of seal blood
- 1 cup of seal fat

ᓄᐊᑦᑎᓚᐅᕐᓗᑎᑦ ᑕᓪᓕᒪᓂᒃ ᐸᐅᓐᓇᓂᒃ, ᐅᕐᑲᐅᔭᖕᒋᑦ, ᐊᒻᒪᓐᓄᑦ ᓱᕋᑦᑎᕐᓗᒋᑦ. ᐃᖑᓚᐅᒻᒨᕐᓗᒋᑦ ᒥᑭᓗᐊᖕᒋᑦᑐᒧᑦ, ᓇᑦᑎᐅᑉ ᐊᐅᖓ ᐃᓚᓕᐅᑎᓗᒍ ᐃᖑᓚᑦᑐᒍ. ᐃᖑᓚᔅᓯᓐᓈᖅ ᓇᑦᑎᐆᑉ ᐅᖅᓯᖓ ᐃᓚᓕᐅᑎᕙᓪᓕᐊᓗᒍ, ᐃᖑᓚᑦᑎᐊᕐᓗᒍ.

After collecting the leaves of five paunnait, roll each stem between your hands until the leaves fall off. Gather the leaves in a bowl and stir in two tablespoons of seal blood. Next, gradually add one cup of fat, mixing very well.

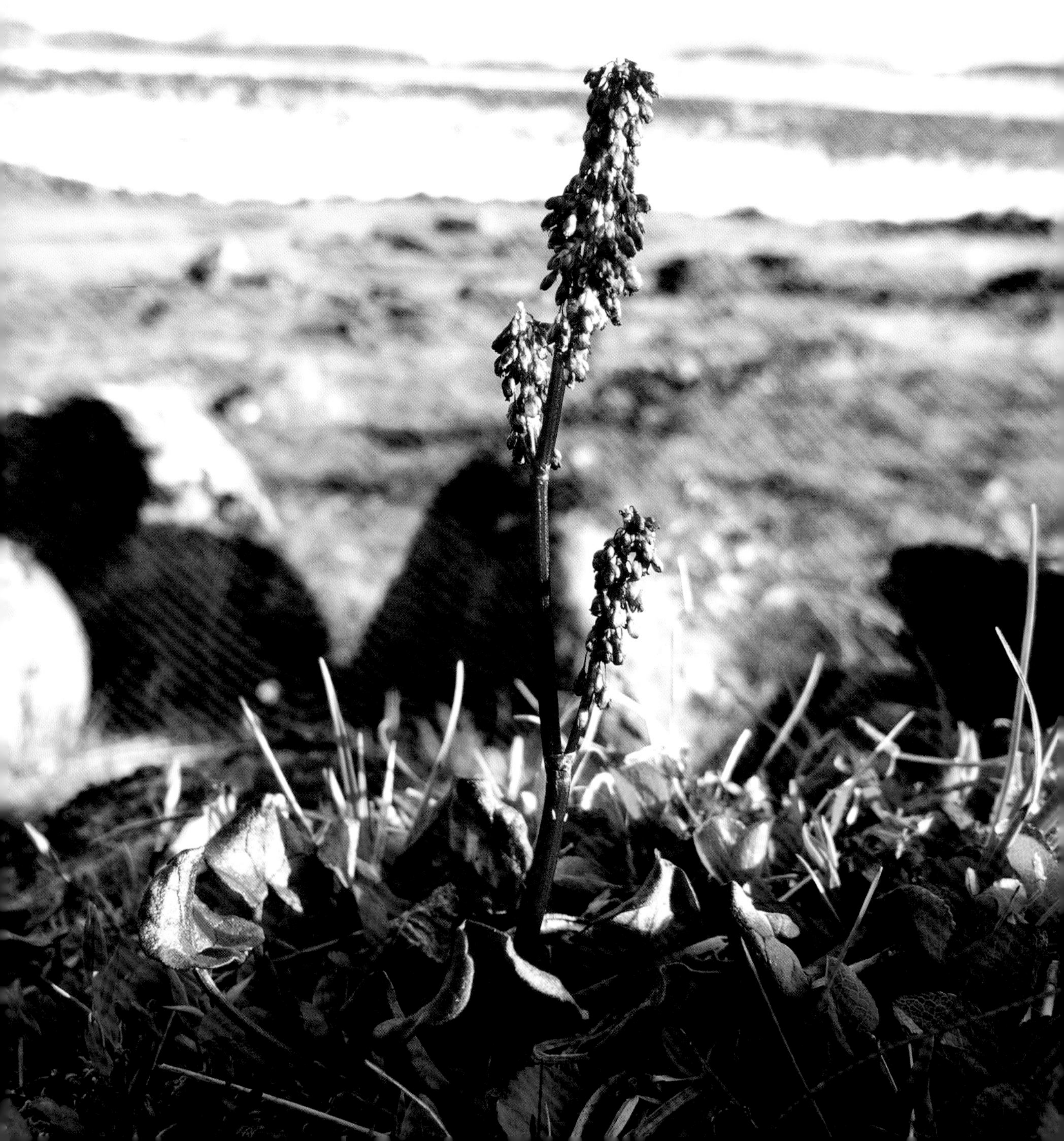

ᖁᖑᓖᑦ
Qunguliit / Mountain Sorrel

ᖁᖑᓖᑦ ᑲᓇᑕᒥ ᓇᒥᑐᐃᓐᓈᓗᒃ ᐱᕈᕇᖑᔪᑦ, ᓄᓇᕗᓯᒫᐸᓗᒻᒥᓪᓗ. ᐅᖅᑯᔭᖕᒋᑦ ᑐᖑᔭᖅᑕᐅᓪᓗᑎᒃ, ᑕᖅᑐᙳᐊᑯᓘᔮᖅᑐᑦ ᑲᑎᒪᓪᓗᑎᑦ ᐱᕈᕇᑦ ᐊᒻᒪᓗ, ᑕᑭᔪᑯᑖᑯᓗᓐᓂᑦ ᐊᐅᐸᓪᓚᓇᑦᑐᓂᒃ ᓇᑲᖅᑲᖅᑐᑎᒃ. ᐅᖅᑯᔭᖕᒋᑦ ᐊᖏᓂᖅᑖᕇᑦ 5–7 ᓯᐊᓐᑎᒦᑐᐸᓗᓐᓂᑦ. ᓇᑲᖕᒋᓪᓚ ᐊᖏᓂᖅᓴᒪᓂᐅᕙᑦᑐᑦ, ᑕᑭᓂᖅᑖᕈᓐᓇᖅᑐᑎᒃ 10–20 ᓯᐊᓐᑎᒦᑐᓂᑦ.

Qunguliit (mountain sorrel) grows in many places throughout Canada, including most parts of Nunavut. It has green, kidney-shaped leaves that grow in clumps and tall, dark red flower stalks that grow up from them. The leaves (known specifically as qunguliit) grow between 5 cm and 7 cm high. The flower stalks (known specifically as *nakait*) are much taller, growing 10 cm to 20 cm high.

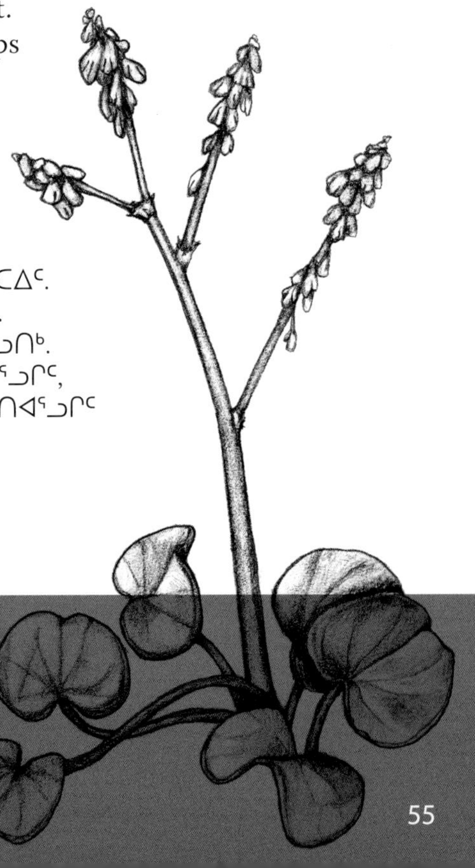

ᕿᓂᕐᓂᐊᕈᕕᐅᓪᓚ, ᐊᐅᐸᕐᓂᖓ ᓇᑲᖓ ᓇᓂᓯᔾᔪᑎᒋᔪᓐᓇᖅᑕᐃᑦ. ᖁᖑᓖᑦ ᒪᒪᕐᓂᖅᐹᑦᑎᐊᖑᕗᑦ ᓂᕆᔭᒃᓴᓂᑦ ᐱᕈᖅᑐᕕᓂᕐᓂᑦ. ᐅᖅᑯᔭᖕᒋᑦ ᓇᑲᖕᒋᓪᓗ ᐃᒃᓯᖅᑲᑦᑎᐊᖅᑐᑎᑦ ᓲᕐᓇᕈᔪᒃᑐᑯᓘᓪᓗᑎᒃ. ᓂᕆᓂᐊᕐᓗᒋᑦ ᖁᖑᓖᑦ, ᓄᐊᑕᑎᑦ ᐊᒃᓴᓪᓗᒋᑦ ᑲᑎᑎᑦᑎᐊᕐᓗᒋᑦ, ᐱᔪᓐᓇᖅᑕᑎᑦ. ᑕᐃᒫ ᓲᕐᓇᖅᑐᑦ ᖃᒃᑭᓐᓇᕐᓂᖅᓴᐃᓪᓗ ᑲᑎᑦᑎᐊᕐᓗᒋᑦ ᒪᒪᖅᑐᑯᓘᓕᖅᑲᑕᖅᑐᑦ. ᖁᖑᓖᑦ ᓂᕿᑦᑎᐊᕚᓗᐃᑦ ᐊᒻᒪ ᐅᖅᑯᑕᐅᓰᖑᓪᓗᑎᑦ ᕙᐃᑕᒥ C-ᖃᓇᖓ.

To find this plant, just look for its red flower stalks. This plant is a treat among all the edible plants. The juicy leaves and stems are tangy with a touch of sweetness. To enjoy this plant, rub a handful of the green leaves and red stems between your palms, squishing them together before you eat them. This combines the sweet and sour juices of the plant to make the most delicious flavour. The leaves and stems are very nutritious and are said to be a good source of vitamin C.

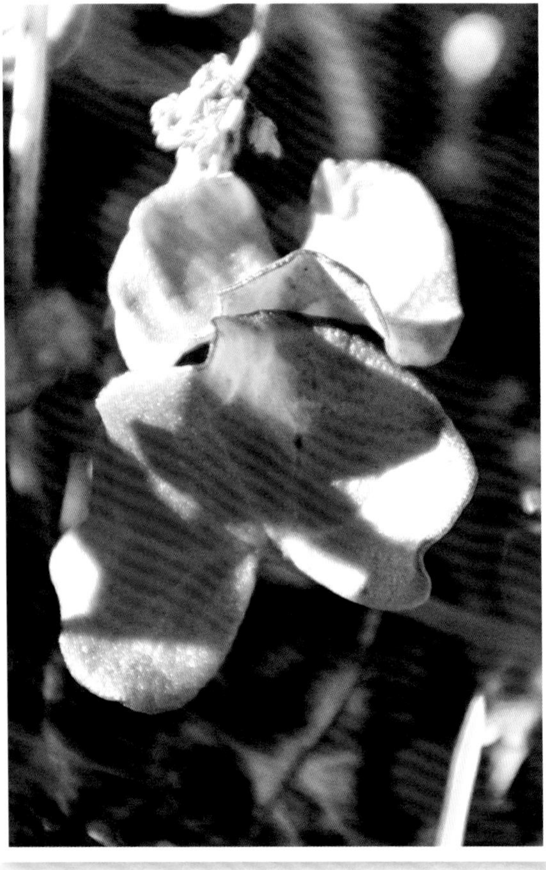

ᓯᑖᓇ ᑲᑦᑐᒃ, ᐅᖅᑲᓕᒫᒐᓕᐅᖅᑑᑉ ᐱᖃᑎᖓ, ᐆᒃᑐᕈᓐᓇᖅᓂᖁᐃᒻᒥᔫᖅ ᐊᒡᒍᒐᑖᑦᑐᕆᑦ ᐅᖅᑲᐅᔭᖕᖏᑦ ᓇᑲᖕᖏᑦᑐ ᑲᔪᖅᒥᑦ ᓯᑲᖅᒥᑦ ᐃᓚᓗᒍ ᓂᕆᓗᓂᑦ ᐃᓚᖅᑎᐊᕚᓘᓂᖁᐃᑦᑐᓂ. ᖁᖑᓖᑦ ᐱᕈᖅᑐᕕᓂᖅᓄᑦ ᑐᖕᖑᔪᖅᑕᓄᑦ ᐃᓚᓕᐅᔾᔭᒃᓴᐅᒻᒥᔪᑦ, ᓲᖅᓗ ᐸᐅᓐᓇᓄᑦ (p. 47) ᐊᒻᒪ ᓯᐅᕋᐅᑉ ᐅᖅᑲᐅᔭᖕᖏᓐᓄᑦ (p. 87).

Celina Kalluk, a friend of the authors, suggests chopping the leaves and flower stalks into small pieces and tossing them with brown sugar to make a delicious side dish. Qunguliit can also be combined with other greens, such as *paunnait* (dwarf fireweed; p. 47) and *siuraup uqaujangit* (seaside bluebells; p. 87).

ᖁᖑᓖᑦ ᐊᐅᔭᓕᒫᖅ ᓂᕆᔭᒃᓴᐅᔪᑦ, ᑭᓯᐊᓂᓕ ᒪᒪᓖᖕᖑᖅᑲᑦᑕᖅᑐᑦ ᐊᐅᔭᐅᑉ ᐃᓱᐸᓗᐊᓂᖅ.

Qunguliit can be eaten all summer long, but it is most nutritious and tasty toward the end of summer.

ᐅᕐᑲᐅᔾᖏᑦ ᓇᑲᖏᓪᓗ
ᐆᑕᒃᓴᐅᒻᒥᔪᑦ. ᐊᕐᕿᓪᓚᒐᔭᖅᑐᑦ
ᑲᔪᕿᔫᓕᕐᓗᑎᓪᓗ ᐊᑯᓂᐅᖏᑦᑐᖅ
ᑎᖅᑎᑦᑐᒦᓚᐅᖅᑎᓪᓗᒋᑦ. ᐅᕐᑲᐅᔾᑦ
ᓇᑲᓪᓗ ᐆᓯᒪᓕᖅᑎᓪᓗᒋᑦ
ᓂᕈᑐᐃᓐᓇᕋᒃᓴᐃᑦ ᐅᖕᖏᓘᓐᓃᑦ
ᓂᕈᓂᐊᖅᑕᓐᓄᑦ ᐃᓚᓕᐅᑎᓗᒋᑦ.
ᓴᙱᓗᐊᖏᑦᑐ ᑎᐱᖓ ᒪᒪᖅᑐᓂᓗ.
ᖃᔪᖓᓗ ᓂᓪᓕᔅᓯᐊᕈᓚᐅᕐᓗᒍ
ᐃᒥᖅᑕᐅᔪᓐᓇᖅᓯᓗᓂ.
ᑖᓐᓇ ᖃᔪᖓ ᓄᑕᕋᕐᓄᑦ
ᐃᒻᒧᒃᓴᖅᑲᖏᑦᑐᓄᑦ ᐱᔭᐅᔪᓐᓇᖅᑐᖅ.
ᐊᑲᐅᓯᔅᓴᐅᑎᐅᒋᓪᓗᓂᑦ
ᐃᒥᖅᑕᐅᔪᓐᓇᕐᒥᔪᑦ
ᓂᕈᔪᒪᖏᑦᑐᐊᓘᓕᖅᑐᓄᑦ.

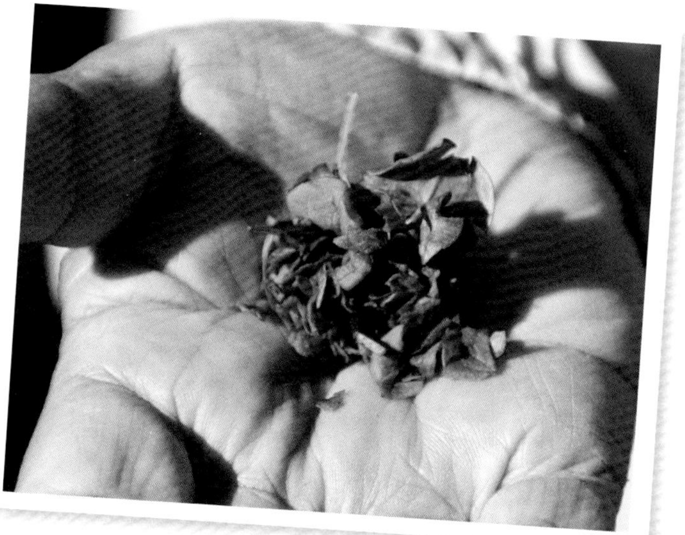

The leaves and flower stalks can also be cooked. They will become tender and light brown when they are boiled briefly. The boiled leaves and stalks can be eaten alone or served as part of a meal. Their flavour will be mild and pleasant.

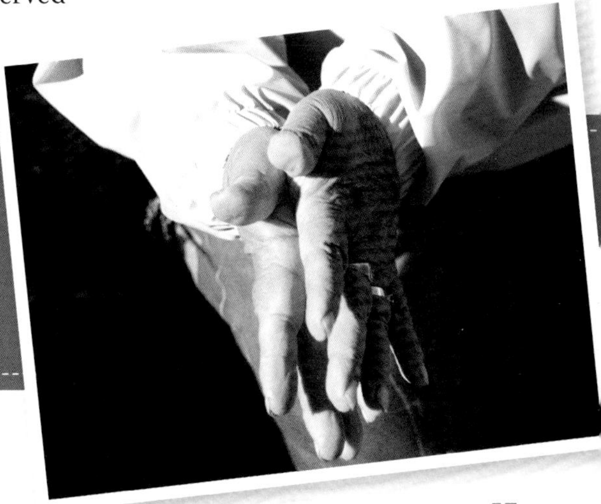

ᐋᓚᓯᐅᑉ ᐊᒃᓴᓕᑦᑕᖏᑦ ᐊᖓᒥᓄᑦ ᖁᖑᓖᑦ
ᐃᒃᓯᓖᑦ ᓲᕐᓇᓕᕇᓂᑦ ᑲᑎᑎᒐᓱᒃᑕᖏᑦ.

Aalasi rubs a handful of qunguliit between her palms to combine the plant's sweet and sour juices.

The clear broth that is left over can be chilled and served as a refreshing drink. This drink may be given to children when milk is not available. It can also be used medicinally to revive a person who has lost their appetite.

ᖁᖑᓕᐅᑉ ᐊᒫᖕᒋᑦ ᒪᒪᖅᑐᑯᓘᒻᒥᔪᑦ ᓂᕿᑦᑎᐊᕙᐅᓪᓗᑎᒃᓗ. ᑭᓯᐊᓂ, ᐆᖃᓯᐅᑎᑦᑕᐃᓕᒃᑭᑦ ᐆᓯᒪᓪᓗᑎᑦ ᒪᒪᕿᓐᓇᐃᓲᖑᒻᒪᑕ. ᓂᕆᓂᐊᕐᓗᒋᓕ, ᐲᔭᕐᓗᒋᑦ ᓂᕆᑐᐃᓐᓇᖁᔪᖅ.

The rhizomes are also tasty and very nutritious. But do not boil them. They are not tasty when cooked. To eat them, just dig them up and enjoy.

ᖁᖑᓖᑦ ᐱᕈᓕᑐᐊᖅᐸᑕ ᓂᕆᔭᒃᓴᐃᑦ, ᑭᓯᐊᓂ ᒪᒪᓛᖑᒋᒍᑦ ᐊᐅᔭᒃᑯᑦ. ᑖᒪᓂᕈᔪᒃ ᑐᖑᑦᑐᕆᑦᑐᑯᓘᕙᑦᑐᑦ ᓂᖅᑭᕆᑦᑐᑎᒃ, ᐅᑭᐊᒃᓴᖓᑐᐊᖅᐸᑦ ᑕᕝᕙ ᐊᐅᐸᕈᔪᒃᓯᓂᐊᕆᓪᓗᑎᑦ.

The leaves and flower stalks can be eaten as soon as they have grown but are most nutritious and flavourful in the late summer. At this time, the leaves will still be green and fleshy, but soon they will turn bright red as the season turns to early autumn.

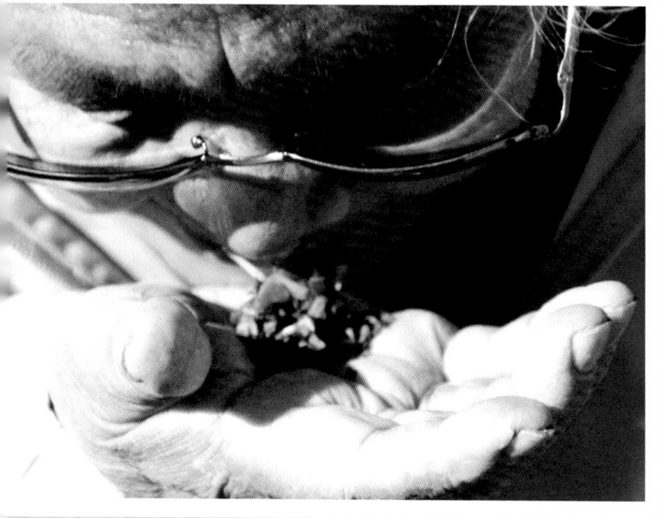

ᐋᓚᓯ ᓇᐃᒪᔪᖅ ᒪᒪᑕᑦᑐᖅ ᖁᖑᓕᓂᑦ. ᖁᖑᓕᑦ ᐃᓅᓕᓴᐅᑎᖅᑲᑦᑎᐊᖅᑐᑦ ᕚᐃᑕᒪᓐ ᑕᓂᑦ.

Aalasi takes in the delicious smell of a handful of qunguliit. Qunguliit is high in vitamin C.

ᖁᖑᓕᐅᑉ ᖃᔪᖕᒐ (ᑎᓯᐃᖕᒐᔪᖅ ᑏᖖᒍᐊᖅ)
Qunguliit Iced Tea

- ᓄᐊᓯᒪᔪᑦ ᐊᒃᑲᓐᓃᓪᓗᐊᖅᑐᑦ ᖁᖑᓖᑦ (ᐊᐃᕿᖃᖕᒋᓪᓗᒋᑦ)
- 5 ᐅᕝᕙᓘᓐᓃᑦ 6 ᐃᕐᖑᓯᑦ ᐃᒪᖅ
- ᓂᓚ

- Several handfuls of fresh qunguliit (with roots removed)
- 5 or 6 cups of water
- Ice

ᑎᖅᑎᑎᓪᓗᒋᑦ ᖁᖑᓖᑦ ᑲᔪᕈᔪᕈᕋᓱᓐᓂᖕᒋᓐᓂᑦ. ᐲᔭᕐᓗᒋᑦ ᖁᖑᓖᑦ (ᓂᕆᓂᐊᑐᐃᓐᓇᕐᓗᒋᑦ) ᐊᒻᒪ ᑎᓯᐃᖅᓯᐊᕆᓗᒍ ᖃᔪᖕᒐ. ᖃᔪᖅ ᓂᓚᓂᑦ ᐃᓗᓪᓕᕐᓗᒍ ᐱᔭᒃᓴᑦᑎᐊᖕᖑᒻᒥᔪᖅ. ᐅᐊᑦᑎᐊᕈᓘᓐᓃᑦ ᐱᖕᒑᕐᓂᐊᕐᓗᒍ ᖁᐊᒃᑯᕕᒻᒦᑎᑕᒃᓴᐅᑎᓪᓗᓂ.

Boil the qunguliit until they turn light brown. Remove the qunguliit (set aside to eat) and then allow the cooking water to cool. Serve the cooking water over ice and enjoy. It can also be refrigerated and saved for later.

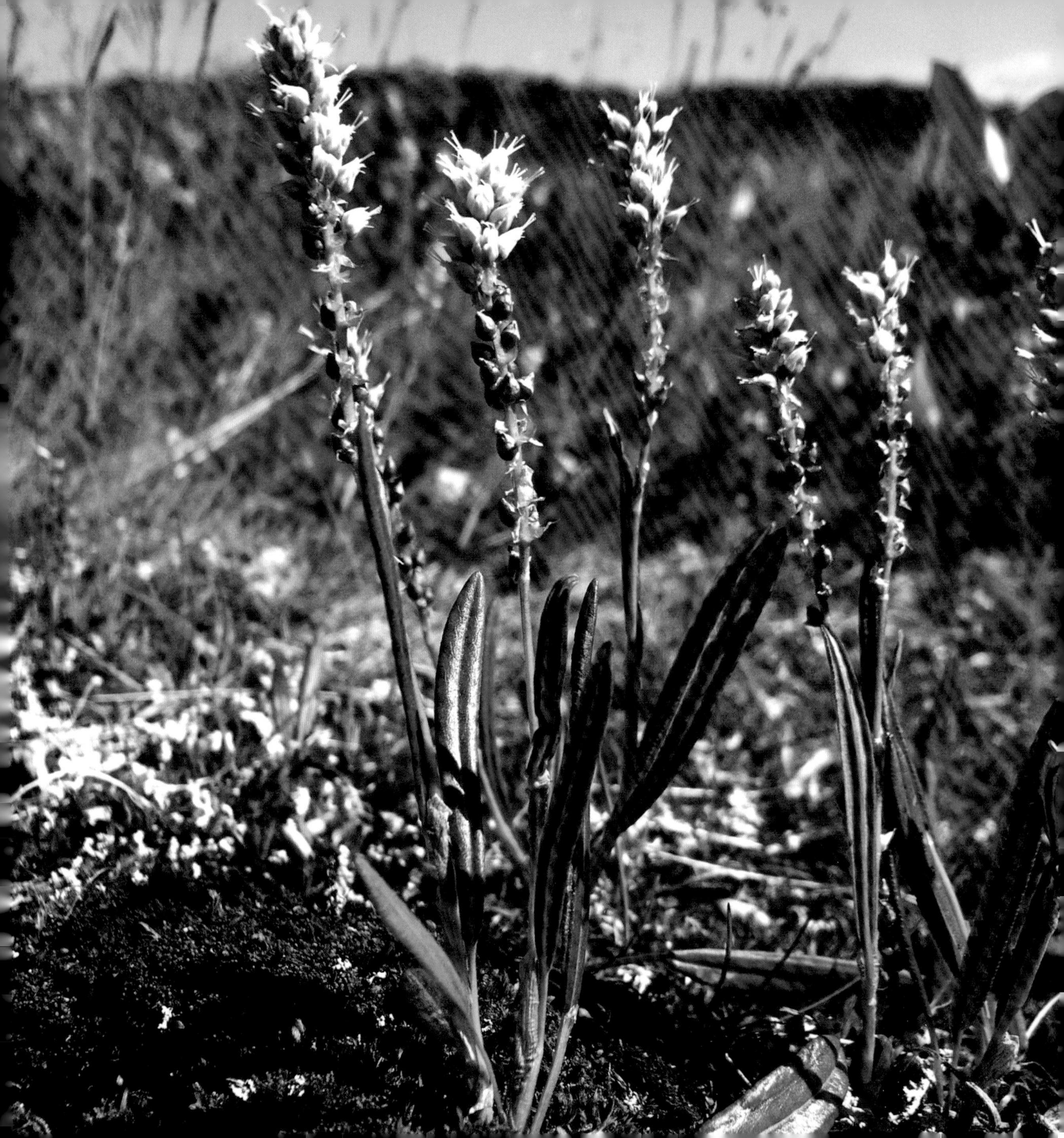

ᓴᐸᖓᕋᓛᙳᐊᑦ ᑐᖅᑕᐃᓪᓗ

Sapangaralaannguat Tuqtaillu / Alpine Bistort

ᓴᐸᖓᕋᓛᙳᐊᑦ, ᐃᓄᒃᑎᑐᑦ ᑐᑭᖃᖅᑐᑦ "ᓴᐸᖓᐅᔮᖅᑐᑦ", ᑖᓐᓇ ᐱᕈᖅᑑᑉ ᓴᖅᑮᔭᕐᓂᖓᓂ ᐅᖃᐅᓯᓕ. ᑐᖅᑕᐃᑦ ᐅᖃᐅᓯᖃᖅᐳᖅ ᐱᕈᖅᑑᑉ ᐃᓚᖓᓂ (ᓇᒃᖓᑕ ᐃᓚᖓ ᓄᓇᑉ ᐊᑖᓂᑦᑐᖅ). ᐅᖃᓕᒫᒐᕐᒥᒃ ᑖᓐᓇ ᓇᓗᓇᐃᖅᓯᒪᔭᕗᑦ ᓴᐸᖓᕋᓛᙳᐊᑦ ᑐᖅᑕᐃᓪᓗ ("ᓴᐸᖓᕋᓛᙳᐊᑦ ᐊᒻᒪᓗ ᑐᖅᑕᐃᑦ") ᐱᔾᔪᑎᒋᓪᓗᒍ ᑕᒪᕐᒥᒃ ᐅᖃᐅᓯᐅᑲᑕᓐᓂᐊᕐᒦᒃ ᐊᑐᓂ.

Sapangaralaannguat, which means "miniature imitation beads" in Inuktitut, refers to the above ground part of alpine bistort. *Tuqtait* refers to its rhizomes. We have called this plant *sapangaralaannguat tuqtaillu* ("sapangaralaannguat and tuqtait") because both parts of the plant are discussed here together.

ᓴᐸᖓᕋᓛᙳᐊᑦ ᑕᑭᔪᑯᑳᑯᓘᕗᑦ, ᖁᑯᖅᑕᓂᒃ ᐱᕈᖅᓯᐊᖅᑐᑎᒃ ᖄᖓᒍᑦ. ᐱᕈᖅᓯᐊᖕᒋᑦ ᒪᐱᓚᐅᖅᑎᓐᓇᒋᑦ, ᓴᐸᖓᑯᓘᔫᖅᑲᑦᑕᖅᑐᑦ, ᐊᐅᐸᖅᑐᑎᒃ. ᑐᖑᔪᖅᑕᐅᓪᓗᑎᒃ ᐅᖃᐅᔭᖕᒋᑦ, ᐊᒥᒃᑐᑯᑳᓘᑦᓗᑎᒃ, ᕿᑦᓕᕈᔫᒃᑐᑎᒃ. ᓇᒃᖓᑕ ᐊᑖᓂ ᐱᕈᖅᑲᑦᑕᖅᑐᑦ. ᓴᐸᖓᕋᓛᙳᐊᑦ ᑕᑭᓂᖅᑲᓕᕈᓐᓇᖅᑐᑦ 25 ᓯᐊᓐᑎᒦᑐᒥᑦ.

Sapangaralaannguat, the above ground part of this plant, has tall green stalks with little white flowers at the top. Before the flowers open, they look like small red beads. The green leaves are long, narrow, and shiny. They grow out from the base of the stalk. Sapangaralaannguat can grow up to 25 cm high.

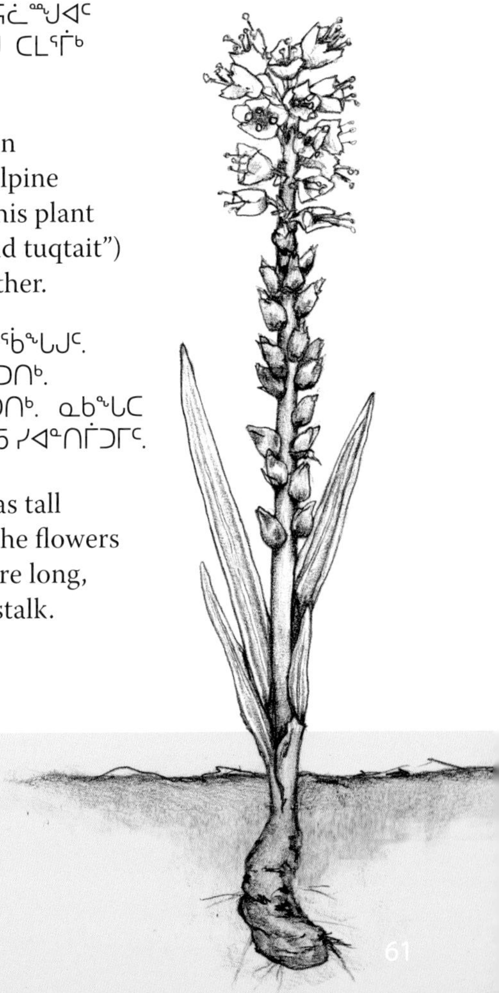

ᑎᓯᔪᑯᓗᐃᑦ “ᓴᐸᖓᙳᐊᑦ” ᓂᕆᔭᒃᓴᑦᑎᐊᖑᔪᑦ ᐱᕈᖅᓯᐊᙳᑕᐅᕐᒋᓐᓂᕐᒋᓐᓂᑦ. ᐅᖃᐅᔾᕐᒋᑦᑐ ᓂᕆᔭᒃᓴᐅᒋᑦᑐᑎᑦ, ᑭᓯᐊᓂ ᓂᕆᔭᐅᒐᓚᕐᒋᑦᑐᑦ ᓂᕆᔪᒥᓇᓗᐊᕐᒋᒻᒪᑕ.

The hard “beads” are enjoyable to eat before they turn into flowers. The leaves are also edible, but they are eaten only if necessary because they have an unpleasant texture.

ᐋᓚᓯ ᐃᖅᑲᐅᒪᔪᖅ ᓂᕈᐊᖅᓯᐊᕐᒍᑦᑐᓂ “ᓴᐸᖓᙳᐊᑦ” ᐱᙳᐊᕆᕙᑦᑐᓂᒋᑦ. ᓄᐊᑕᐅᔪᓐᓇᖅᑐᑦ ᐊᐃᑦ ᐱᕆᓯᒪᓗᒍ ᑕᒪᐅᖓ ᐱᕆᓐᓂᖓᓄᑦ, ᖃᖓᑐᐃᓐᓇ ᐅᑦᑑᑉ ᐃᓗᐊᓂ ᓂᕐᒪᑲᑕᓐᓂᐊᕐᓗᒋᑦ. ᓴᐸᖓᕋᓛᙳᐊᑦ ᓄᐊᑦᑐᒋᑦ ᖃᑦᑐᓈᖅᑕᒧᑦ ᕿᑲᑦᑐᒋᑦ “ᑎᒍᒥᐊᒐᒃ” ᑎᒍᒥᐊᖅᑳᑕᓚᐊᕆᔭᒃᓴᐅᒻᒥᔪᑦ. ᑎᒍᒥᐊᒐᒃ ᐊᔅᓴᑦᑐᒍ ᐊᒡᒐᕝᕕᑦ ᐃᑎᒪᖓᓄᑦ.

Aalasi recalls playing with the beads as a young girl. They can be collected in the pouch of a sleeve folded up at the wrist and eaten throughout the day. The beads can also be collected and tied into a small sack to create a soothing “stress ball.” Roll the sack in the palm of your hand.

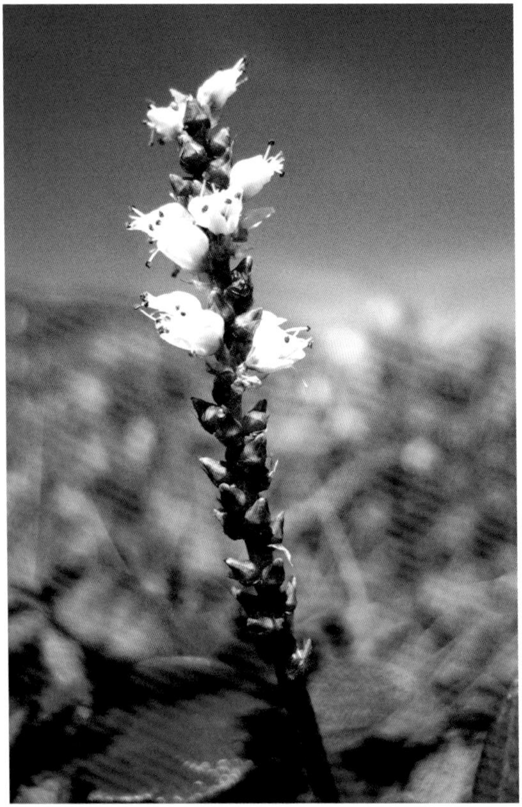

ᓴᐸᖓᕋᓛᙳᐊᑦ (“ᓴᐸᖓᐅᔫᖅᑐᑦ ᒥᑭᑦᑐᑯᓗᐃᑦ) ᐊᑎᖅᑐᑎᖅᖅᑐᑦ ᒥᑭᑦᑐᑯᓗᐃᑦ, ᐊᐅᐸᖅᑐᑦ “ᓴᐸᖓᙳᐊᕐᒋᓐᓄᑦ” ᐱᕈᖅᓯᐊᙳᕐᓂᑦ ᐊᐅᔭᐅᑉ ᕿᑎᐸᓗᐊᓂᑦ.

Sapangaralaannguat (“miniature imitation beads”) is named for its tiny red “beads” that turn into flowers mid-season.

ᑐᖅᑕᐃᑦ, ᓇᑲᙵᑕ ᐃᓚᙵ, ᒪᒪᖅᑐᒻᒪᕆᐅᔪᑦ ᓂᕿᑦᑎᐊᕙᐅᓪᓗᑎᓪᓗ. ᐃᓗᒥᑦ ᓴᓗᒻᒪᐃᑦᑎᐊᕈᓐᓇᕐᒥᔪᑦ. ᑎᓯᓂᙵ ᑎᐱᙵᓗ ᖃᖅᑯᐊᒐᑎᑑᐸᓗᒃᑐᑦ. ᑐᖅᑕᐃᑦ ᐳᑐᐃᓐᓇᖅᓴᐅᕗᑦ.

Tuqtait, the rhizomes, are very tasty and nutritious. They also cleanse the digestive system. Their texture and taste are similar to almonds. Tuqtait can be enjoyed fresh from the ground. Use a small shovel or your fingers to dig them up. Detach them from the rest of the plant and clean off the small white stems with your fingernail.

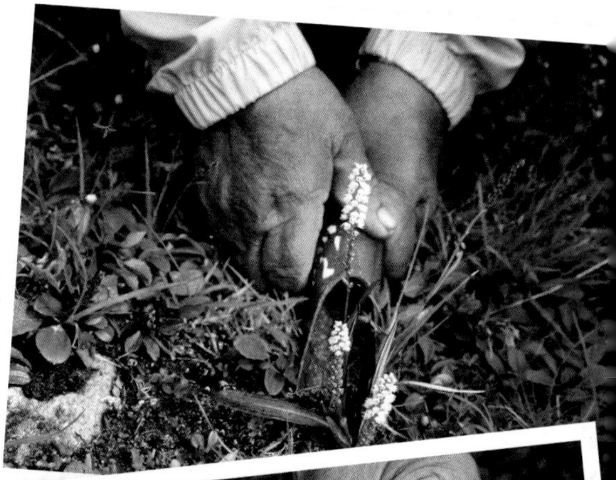

ᐆᓯᒪᓪᓗᑎᓪᓚ, ᑐᖅᑕᐃᑦ ᐊᕿᑦᑐᑯᓘᕗᑦ, ᓲᕐᓗᑕ ᑖᑏᓯᖁᓛᑎᑐᑦ. ᐆᓯᒪᓗᑎᑦ ᓂᖓᓂᐊᕈᖕᕕᒋᑦ, ᑎᖅᑎᑎᕐᑯᔪᑦ 5–10 ᐃᑲᕐᖂᕿᓯᐸᓗᓐᓂᑦ, ᐊᕿᑦᑕᓇᓲᓐᓂᖕᒋᓐᓂᑦ.

When cooked, tuqtait are mild and soft, like very tiny potatoes. To enjoy them cooked, boil them until they are tender, about 5 to 10 minutes.

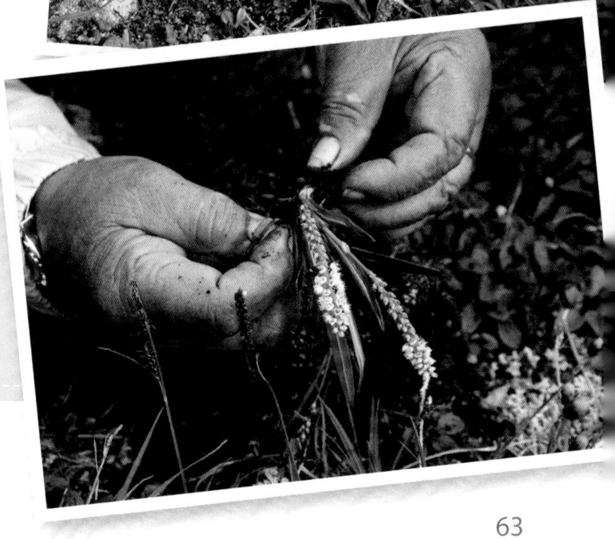

ᐋᓚᓯ ᓄᐊᑦᑎᑎᓪᓗᒍ ᑐᖅᑕᓂᑦ (ᐊᒫᖕᒋᓐᓂᒃ), ᖃᓗᕋᖅᑐᓂᒋᑦ ᐲᔭᖅᑐᓂᒋᑦ ᓴᐸᖓᕋᓛᙳᐊᓂᑦ (ᓄᓇᐅᑉ ᖄᖓᓃᓐᓂᖓ ᐱᕈᖅᑑᑉ).

Aalasi harvests tuqtait (the rhizomes), digging them up and detaching them from the sapangaralaannguat (the above ground part of the plant).

ᑐᖅᑕᐃᑦ ᐊᒃᑐᒐᓛᓪᓗᒋᑦ ᓂᕿᓄᑦ ᐃᓚᒃᓴᑦᑎᐊᕙᕆᕗᑦ. ᐊᒃᑐᒐᓛᒃᓯᒪᔪᑦ ᐸᓚᐅᒑᓕᐊᒧᑦ ᐃᓚᓕᐅᑎᔭᒃᓴᐅᕆᕗᑦ ᐆᓚᐅᖏᓐᓂᕐᓂᑦ ᐸᓚᐅᒑᖅ. ᐃᓚᓕᐅᑎᒐᒃᓴᐅᕆᕗᑦ ᑲᑎᑕᐹᓄᑦ ᐅᖅᑲᐅᔭᓄᑦ ᑐᖑᔪᖅᑕᓄᑦ ᐆᒃᑑᑎᕆᓗᒍ, ᑲᑎᓯᒪᔪᑦ ᖁᖑᓖᑦ (p. 55) ᐸᐅᓐᓇᐃᑦᑐ (p. 47) ᒪᒪᖅᑐᐊᓘᕗᑦ ᑐᖅᑕᓂᒃ ᐃᓚᓯᒪᓪᓗᒋᑦ. ᑐᖅᑕᐃᑦ ᑎᓯᓂᖅᓴᒻᒪᕆᐅᖁᒍᕕᒋᑦ ᒪᒪᕐᓂᖅᓴᐅᓗᓂᓗ, ᐅᓪᓗᓕᒫᖅ ᓂᓪᓕᓇᖅᑐᒥᒃ ᐃᒫᓃᑎᖁᔪᖅ ᓂᕆᓚᐅᖏᓐᓂᕐᓂᑦ.

Tuqtait can also be used as a seasoning for other foods by chopping them into small pieces. The pieces can be added to the batter of bannock before baking or frying it. They can also be added to greens. For example, a mixture of *qunguliit* (mountain sorrel; p. 55) and *paunnait* (dwarf fireweed; p. 47) is delicious topped with tuqtait. To make tuqtait even crunchier, soak them in cold water for a day before eating.

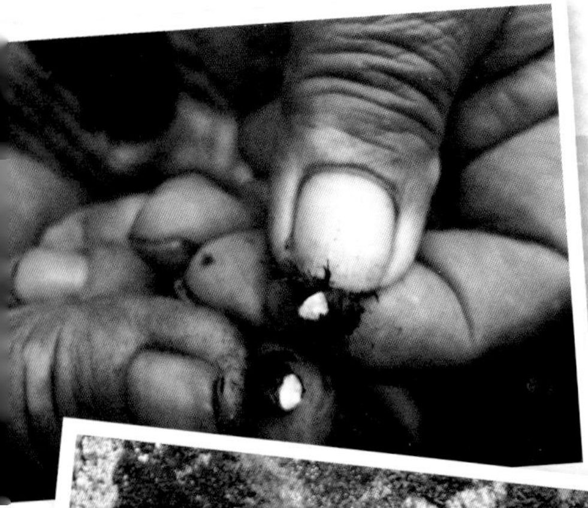

ᐋᓚᓯ ᑐᖅᑕᒥᑦ ᖁᐱᓯᑎᓪᓗᒍ. ᑐᖅᑕᐃᑦ ᖃᖅᑯᐊᒐᖅᑎᑐᑦ ᒪᒪᖅᑎᕆᔪᑦ ᑎᓯᕈᔪᒃᑐᑯᓘᓪᓗᑎᓪᓗ.

Aalasi breaks open tuqtait. Tuqtait have a mild almond flavour and an enjoyable crunch.

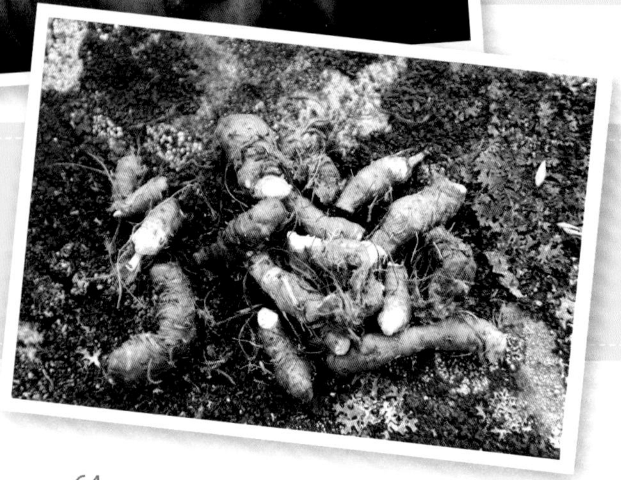

ᑐᖅᑕᐃᑦ ᓂᕿᑦᑎᐊᕚᓗᐃᑦ. ᐆᓯᒪᖏᓪᓗᑎᒃ ᓂᕆᔭᒃᓴᐃᑦ ᖃᖅᑯᐊᒐᖅᑎᑐᑦ, ᐆᑦᑎᓗᒋᓪᓗᓐᓃᑦ, ᓲᕐᓗ ᑖᑎᓯᕋᓛᑎᑐᑦ.

Tuqtait are very nutritious. They can be enjoyed raw, like nuts, or cooked, like tiny potatoes.

ᑐᖅᑕᖅ ᐃᖅᑲᓗᕕᓂᓕᒃ ᐸᐅᖅᖕᒐᐃᓪᓗ
Char Salad with Tuqtait and Paurngait (Crowberries)

- 6 ᑐᖅᑕᐃᑦ, ᐊᒃᑐᒐᓛᔅᓯᒪᔫᑦ
- 1 ᓇᑉᐸᖅ ᐃᖅᑲᓗᕕᓂᖅ (2–3 ᐃᓐᑦᓯᔅ ᓯᓚᓐᓂᓚᒃ), ᓴᐅᓃᔭᖅᓯᒪᔪᖅ ᐊᒥᖅᑲᖃᓂᓗ ᐆᔪᖅ
- 1 ᐃᖅᖕᒍᓯᖅ ᐸᐅᖅᖕᒐᐃᑦ (p. 68) ᐊᓯᖕᒋᑦ ᓘᓐᓂᑦ ᐸᐅᖅᖕᒐᑐᐃᓐᓇᐃᑦ
- 2 ᐊᓘᑎᑯᔅᓯᒃ ᐄᔭᖅᓂᕈᑎ, ᐱᑕᖅᑲᕈᓂ ᑭᓯᐊᓂ (ᐊᓯᖕᒋᑦ ᓘᓐᓃᑦ ᐅᖅᓱᑐᐃᓐᓇᖅ, ᓇᑦᑎᐅᑦ ᓘᓐᓃᑦ ᐅᖅᓱᖅᖕᒐᓂ)

- 6 tuqtait, chopped into small pieces
- 1 section of a char (about 2 to 3 inches thick), boiled with all skin and bones removed
- 1 cup of *paurngait* (crowberries; p. 68) or other berries
- 2 tablespoons of mayonnaise, if available (or other fat, such as seal fat)

ᐃᖅᑲᓗᕕᓂᖅ ᓵᓘᖅᑐᒍ ᐃᖕᒍᓚᓪᓗᒍ ᓱᕿᑦᑎᖅᑐᓂ. ᐃᓚᓕᐅᑎᓗᒋᑦ ᑐᖅᑕᐃᑦ ᐄᔭᖅᓂᕈᑎᓗ ᐊᒻᒪ ᐃᖕᒍᓚᑦᑎᐊᖅᓗᒋᑦ. ᐸᐅᖅᓇᐃᑦ ᐃᓚᓕᐅᑎᑎᖅᒥᓗᒋᑦ, ᖅᑲᐅᖅᑕᐃᓕᒪᓗᒋᑦ ᐃᖕᒍᓚᒃᑲᓐᓂᖅᓗᒋᑦ. ᐆᓇᕈᔫᓐᓂᖕᒐᓂᑦ ᓂᕆᔭᐅᔭᕆᐊᓕᒃ.

Place the boiled char in a bowl and break it into flakes. Add the tuqtait and mayonnaise and mix well. Add the berries, mixing gently so they are not squished. Serve warm.

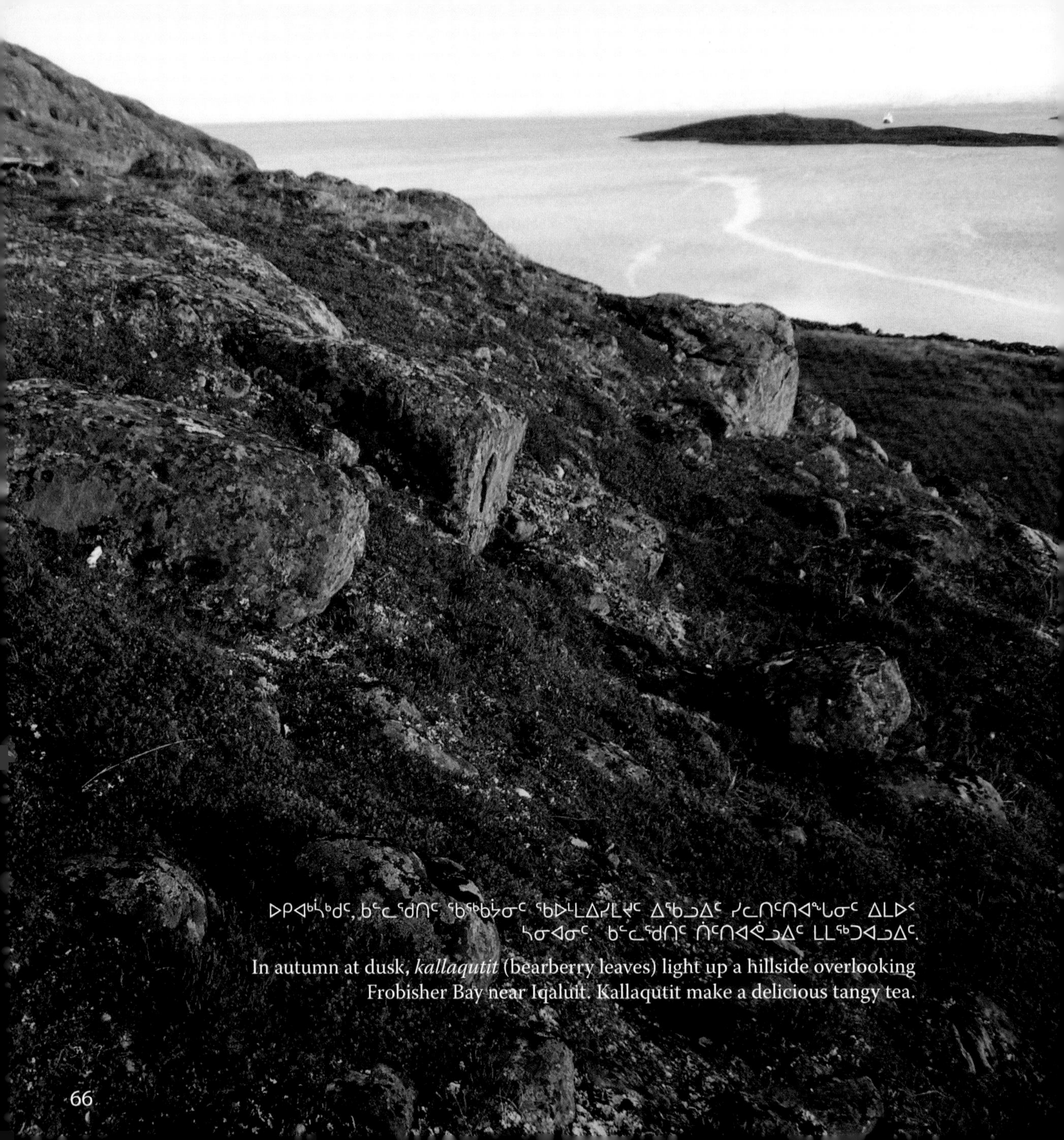

ᐅᑭᐊᒃᓵᒃᑯᑦ, ᑲᓪᓚᖁᑎᑦ ᖃᖅᑳᔾᓂᑦ ᖃᐅᒻᒪᐃᓯᒪᔪᑦ ᐃᖃᓗᐃᑦ ᓯᓚᑎᑦᑎᐊᖓᓂᑦ ᐃᒪᐅᑉ
ᓴᓂᐊᓂᑦ. ᑲᓪᓚᖁᑏᑦ ᑏᑦᑎᐊᕚᓗᐃᑦ ᒪᒪᖅᑐᐊᓗᐃᑦ.

In autumn at dusk, *kallaqutit* (bearberry leaves) light up a hillside overlooking Frobisher Bay near Iqaluit. Kallaqutit make a delicious tangy tea.

ᐸᐅᕐᖓᐃᑦ ᐊᔾᔨᒌᖏᑦᑐᑦ
Paurngait Ajjigiingittut / Berry Plants

ᐊᐅᔭᐅᑉ ᕿᑎᓪᓚᓇᖓᓂᑦ ᓇᒥᑐᐃᓐᓈᓗᒃ ᐸᐅᕐᖓᑯᓗᖕᓂᑦ ᐅᑭᐅᖅᑕᖅᑐᖅ ᐱᕈᕝᕕᐅᓲᖑᔪᖅ. ᐱᖕᒐᓲᔫᓪᓚ ᓇᑐᓇᐃᕐᓂᐊᖅᑕᔪᑦ ᐅᕙᓂ: ᐸᐅᕐᖓᐃᑦ ᐸᐅᕐᖓᖁᑎᓪᓗ, ᑲᓪᓚᐃᑦ ᑲᓪᓚᖅᑯᑎᓪᓗ, ᐊᒻᒪᓗ ᑭᒍᑕᖏᕐᓇᑦ ᓇᖁᑎᓪᓗ. ᐸᐅᕐᖓᐃᑦ ᐊᔾᔨᒌᖏᑦᑐᑦ ᑖᒃᑯᐊᑦ ᐋᓚᓯᐅᑉ ᖃᐅᔨᒪᒌᓂᕙᐃᑦ.

In late summer, many regions of the Arctic are rich with juicy berries. Three different berry plants are described here: *paurngait paurngaqutillu* (crowberry; p. 68), *kallait kallaqutillu* (bearberry; p. 72), and *kigutangirnait naqutillu* (blueberry; p. 75). These are the berry plants with which Aalasi is most familiar.

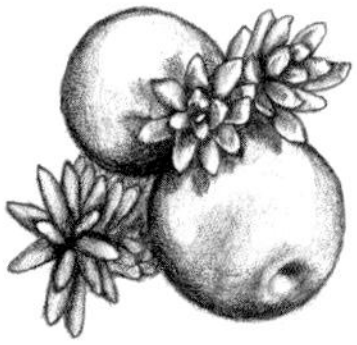

ᐸᐅᕐᖓᐃᑦ ᐸᐅᕐᖓᖁᑎᓪᓗ

Paurngait Paurngaqutillu / Crowberry

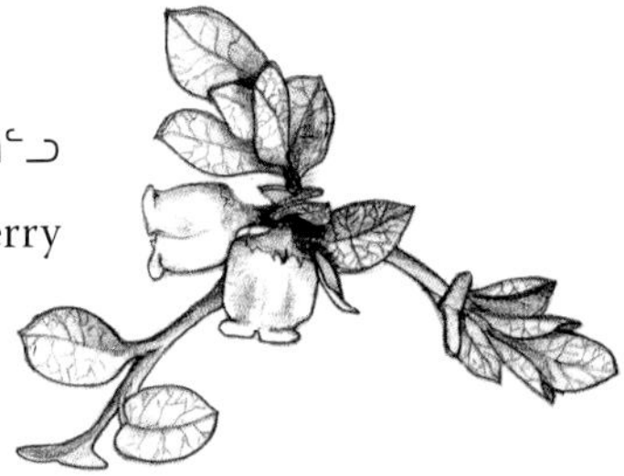

ᑭᒍᑕᖏᕐᓇᐃᑦ ᓇᖁᑎᓪᓗ

Kigutangirnait Naqutillu / Blueberry

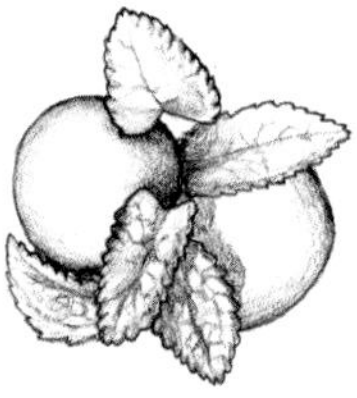

ᑲᓪᓚᐃᑦ ᑲᓪᓚᖁᑎᓪᓗ

Kallait Kallaqutillu / Bearberry

ᐸᐅᕐᖓᐃᑦ ᐸᐅᕐᖓᖁᑎᓪᓗ

Paurngait Paurngaqutillu / Crowberry

ᐃᓄᒃᑎᑐᑦ ᐸᐅᕐᖓᐃᑦ (ᐊᑕᐅᓯᐅᓪᓗᓂ: ᐸᐅᕐᖓᖅ) ᐸᐅᕐᖓᓂᑦ ᐱᕈᖅᑐᓂᑦ ᐅᖃᐅᓯᖅᑲᖅᐳᖅ ᐊᒻᒪᓗ ᐸᐅᕐᖓᖁᑎᑦ ᐅᖃᐅᓴᖏᓐᓂᑦ ᐱᕈᕐᕕᖏᓐᓂᑦ ᐅᖃᐅᓯᖅᑲᖅᑐᑦ. ᐅᕙᓂᓕ ᑕᐃᑲᑕᑉᐸᕗ ᐸᐅᕐᖓᐃᑦ ᐸᐅᕐᖓᖁᑎᓪᓗ.

In Inuktitut, *paurngait* (singular: *paurngaq*) refers to the berries of this plant and *paurngaqutit* refers to the leaves. Here, we refer to this plant generally as *paurngait paurngaqutillu* ("paurngait and paurngaqutit").

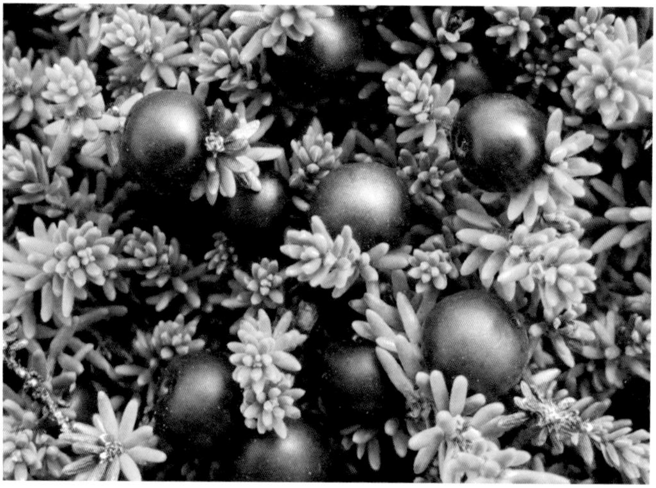

ᐸᐅᕐᖓᐃᑦ ᐸᐅᕐᖓᕐᑯᑎᓪᓗ ᐱᑕᕐᑲᒐᔪᑦᑐᑦ ᓄᓇᓕᖕᓂᑦ ᓄᓇᕗᒻᒥᑦ (ᐱᑕᕐᑲᓗᐊᙱᑦᑐᑦ ᑭᓯᐊᓂ ᕿᑎᕐᒥᐅᓂᑦ). ᐃᓕᓴᕆᔭᕐᓂᖅᐸᑦ ᐅᕐᑲᐅᔭᖕᒥᑦ ᑐᖕᒍᑦᑐᕆᐅᔭᐃᓐᓇᕐᒪᑕ, ᒥᖅᑯᑎᐅᔮᖅᑐᑎᑦ ᑲᔫᓂᕐᒪᓂᒃ ᓇᑲᕐᒪᓃᙶᖅᑐᑦ. ᓇᑲᕐᒥᑦ ᐱᕈᕐᑲᑦᑕᖅᑐᑦ ᓯᓕᑦᑐᑎᒃ ᐊᒻᒪᓗ ᓂᒐᕕᐅᖅᑲᔪᑯᓘᓪᓗᑎᒃ ᐊᒻᒪ 15 ᓯᐊᓐᑎᒦᑐᒥᑦ ᐊᖏᓂᖅᓴᐅᓕᕈᓐᓇᖏᑦᑐᑦ. ᐃᔾᔨᓂᑦ ᐊᒥᐊᓕᓐᓂᑦ ᐱᕈᖅᓯᐊᑖᑲᐃᓐᓇᕐᑲᑦᑕᖅᑐᑦ ᑭᓯᐊᓂ ᕿᓚᒥᑯᓗᒃ (ᕿᓂᑲᐅᖅᑐᖕᒋᒃᑯᕕᒋᑦ, ᑕᑯᙱᑕᐃᓐᓇᕐᓂᐊᖅᐸᑎᑦ!). ᐸᐅᕐᖓᐃᑦ ᐊᒻᒪᓗᑭᔮᖑᕗᑦ ᐃᒃᓯᕐᑲᑦᑎᐊᖅᑐᑎᑦ. ᐱᕈᓕᔮᖅᑐᑎᑦ ᑐᖑᔪᖅᑕᐅᕐᑲᑦᑕᖅᑐᑦ ᑕᕝᕙ ᕿᕐᓂᖅᓯᑕᕆᑦᑐᑎᑦ ᓂᕆᔭᒃᓴᐅᓕᖄᕐᒪᑕ ᐊᐅᔭᒃᑯᑦ.

Paurngait paurngaqutillu is common around many communities in Nunavut (although somewhat less common in the Kitikmeot). It is easily recognizable by its evergreen leaves, which look like short needles sticking out from the brown stems. The stems grow into thick tangles on the ground and are usually less than 15 cm high. The tiny purple flowers appear very briefly in early spring (if you don't look at the right time, you will miss them!). The paurngait are round and juicy. They are green when they first appear and then turn black and shiny when they are ripe in the late summer.

ᔪᓚᐃ ᐱᒋᐊᕐᓂᖓᓂᑦ, ᐸᐅᕐᖓᐃᑦ ᑖᒃᑯᐊ ᐱᕈᓈᙱᑦᑑᒐᓗᐊᑦ, ᑭᓯᐊᓂ ᒪᒪᖅᑐᑰᓕᖅᑐᑦ ᐃᒃᓯᕐᑲᑦᑎᐊᖅᑐᑎᑦᓗ.

In early July, these paurngait are not ripe yet, but they already taste pleasant and refreshing.

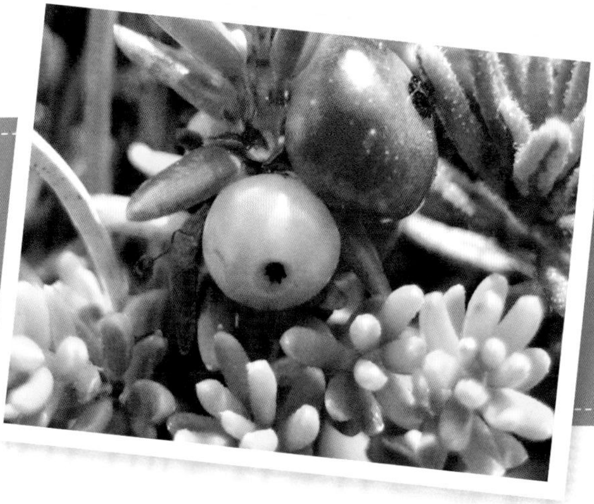

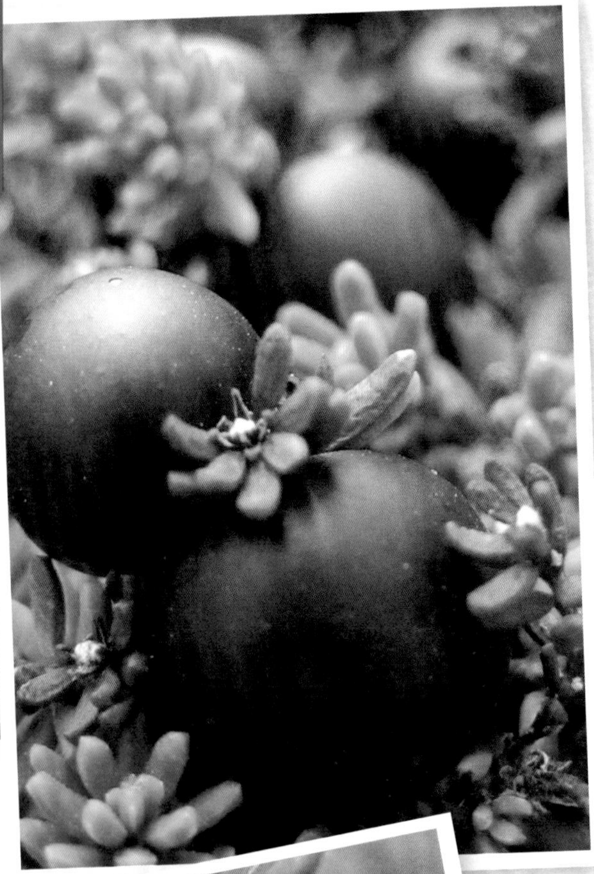

ᓴᐅᓈᖕᒋᑦ ᖃᒃᑭᓐᓇᖅᑐᑦ, ᐸᐅᖕᒐᐃᑦ ᐳᕙᓚᔪᑦ ᓲᕐᓇᖅᑐᑯᓗᐃᑦ.

While the seeds are slightly bitter, the meat of ripe paurngait is tangy and sweet.

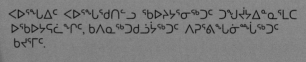

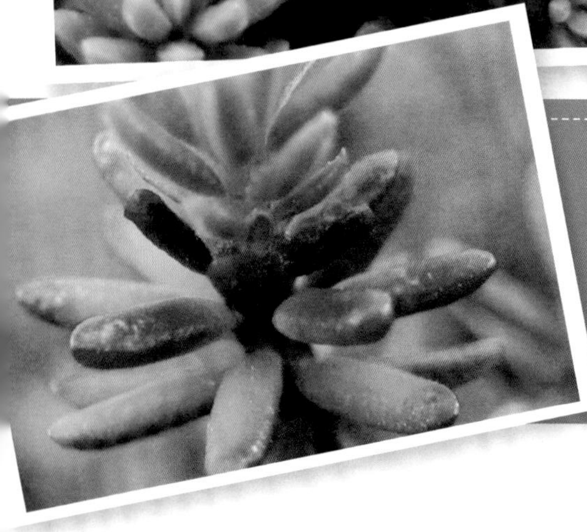

ᐸᐅᖕᒐᐃᑦ ᐸᐅᖕᒐᕐᑯᑎᓪᓗ ᖃᐅᔨᓴᕐᓂᖅᑐᑦ ᑐᖕᒍᕚᔭᐃᓐᓇᕐᒪᑕ ᐅᖃᐅᔭᕐᑖᖕᒋᑦ, ᑲᐱᓇᖅᑐᑯᓘᔭᖅᑐᑦ ᐱᕈᕐᕕᖕᒐᓃᖖᒑᖅᑐᑦ ᑲᔪᕐᒥᑦ.

Paurngait paurngaqutillu is easily recognizable by its evergreen leaves, which look like short needles sticking out from the brown stems.

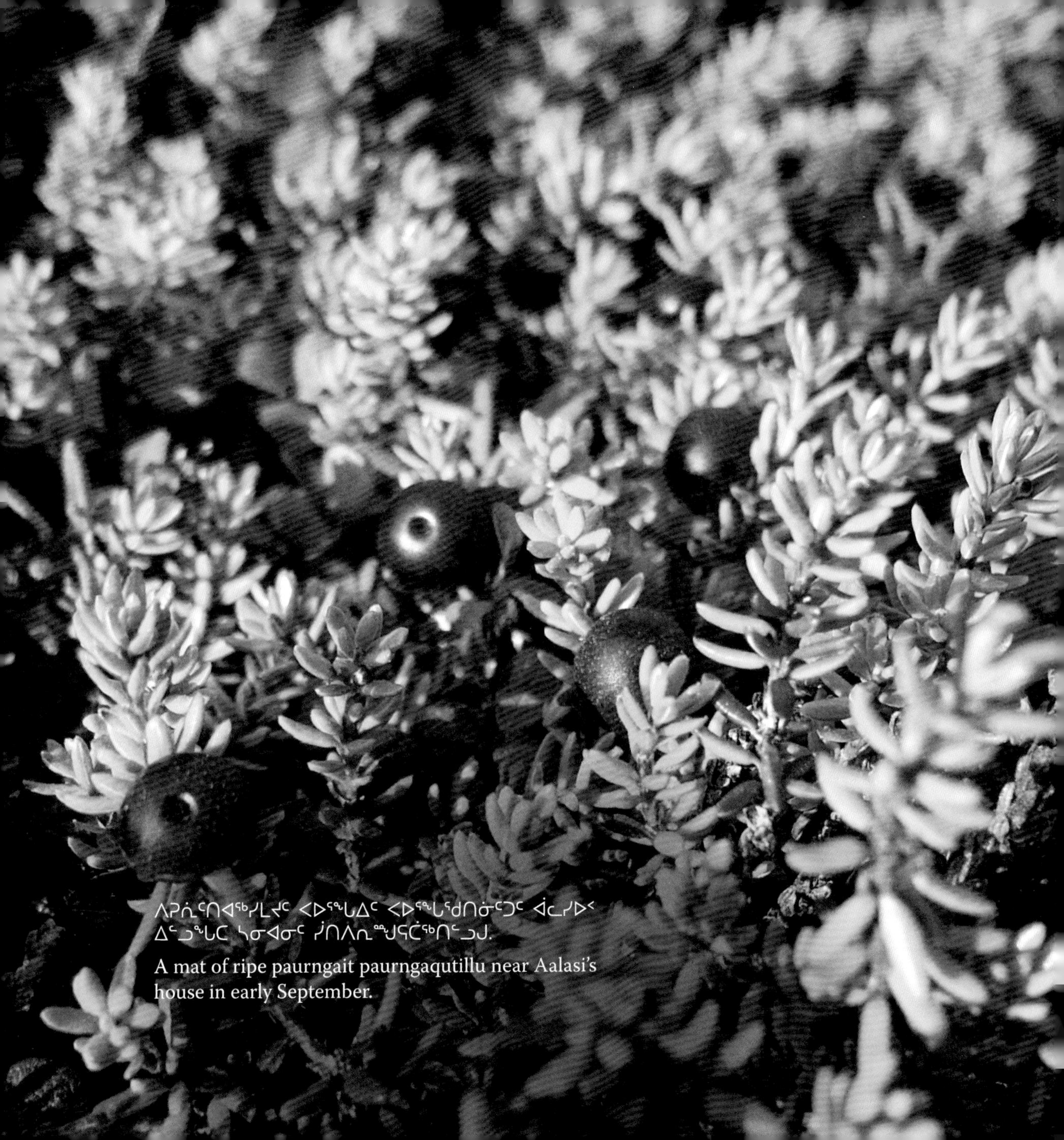

ᐱᕈᓅᕐᑎᐊᖅᓯᒪᔪᑦ ᐸᐅᖕᖓᐃᑦ ᐸᐅᖕᖓᕐᑯᑎᓐᓂᑦᑐᑦ ᐋᓚᓯᐅᑉ
ᐃᓪᓗᖓᑕ ᓴᓂᐊᓂᑦ ᓲᑎᐱᓇᙵᕋᑖᖅᑎᓪᓗᒍ.

A mat of ripe paurngait paurngaqutillu near Aalasi's house in early September.

ᑲᓪᓚᐃᑦ ᑲᓪᓚᖁᑎᓪᓗ
Kallait Kallaqutillu / Bearberry

ᐃᓄᒃᑎᑐᑦ, ᑲᓪᓚᐃᑦ (ᐊᑕᐅᓯᐅᓪᓗᓂ: ᑲᓪᓚᒃ) ᐸᐅᖖᒐᖏᓐᓂᑦ ᐅᖃᐅᓯᖃᖅᐳᖅ ᐊᒻᒪ ᑲᓪᓚᖁᑎᑦ ᐅᖃᐅᔭᖏᓐᓂᑦ ᐱᕈᕐᕕᖏᓐᓂᑦ ᐅᖃᐅᓯᖃᖅᑐᑎᑦ. ᐅᕙᓂᓕ ᑕᐃᑲᑕᓐᓂᐊᖅᑕᕗᑦ ᑲᓪᓚᐃᑦ ᑲᓪᓚᖁᑎᓪᓗ.

In Inuktitut, *kallait* (singular: *kallak*) refers to the fruit and *kallaqutit* refers to the leaves of the plant. Here, we refer to the plant generally as *kallait kallaqutillu* ("kallait and kallaqutit").

ᑲᓪᓚᐃᑦ ᑲᓪᓚᖁᑎᓪᓗ ᐱᑕᖃᒐᔪᑦᑐᒻᒪᕇᑦ ᕿᑭᖅᑕᓂ, ᑭᕙᓪᓕᕐᒥᓗ ᓄᓇᐃᑦ ᐃᓚᖏᓐᓂᑦ, ᐊᒻᒪᓗ ᕿᑎᕐᒥᐅᓂ. ᑲᓪᓚᐃᑦ ᑲᓪᓚᖁᑎᓗᓪ ᓇᓗᓇᖏᑦᑎᐊᖅᑐᑦ ᑕᒻᒪᐅᑕᐅᔪᓐᓇᕐᑎᓪᓗ ᑭᒍᑕᖏᕐᓇᐃᑦ ᓇᖁᑎᖏᓐᓂᓪᓗ. ᐅᖃᐅᔭᖏᑕ ᑭᓪᓕᖏᑦ ᑐᑭᓕᐊᑦᑎᐊᖏᒻᒪᑕ (ᑭᒍᑕᖏᕐᓇᐃᑦ ᓇᖁᑎᓪᓗ ᑐᑭᓕᐊᑦᑎᐊᖅᑐᓂᑦ ᐅᖃᐅᔭᖃᕐᒪᑕ). ᐅᖃᐅᔭᖏᑦ ᑕᑯᔅᓴᐅᑦᑎᐊᖅᑐᑦ

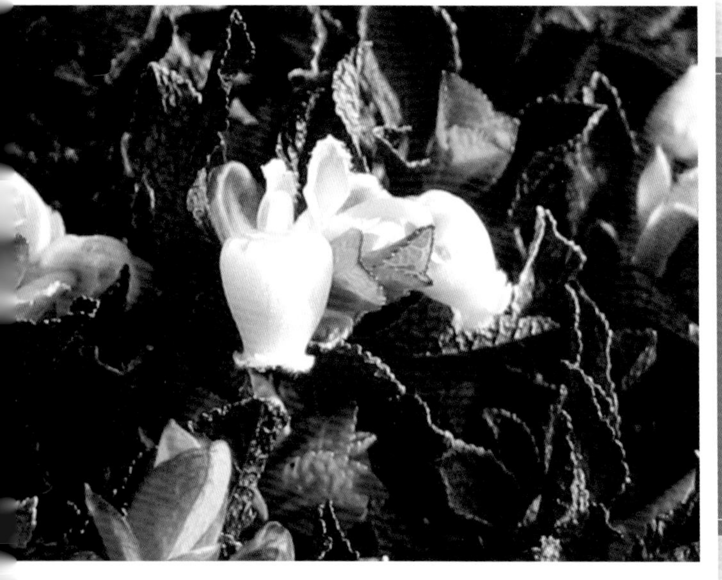

ᐱᕈᖅᓯᐊᕋᓛᑦ ᓄᕗᐊᓃᑦᑐᑦ ᑲᓪᓚᐃᑦ ᑲᓪᓚᖁᑏᓪᓗ ᓴᖅᑭᔮᑲᐃᓐᓇᑐᐃᓐᓇᖃᑦᑕᖅᑐᑦ ᐊᐅᔭᐅᓚᓵᖅᑎᓪᓗᒍ. ᐅᕙᓂ ᐊᔾᔨᖖᒍᐊᒥᑦ ᐅᖃᐅᔭᖏᑦ ᑐᖑᔪᖅᑐᑦ ᐊᕐᕌᓂᓴᕐᓃᖅᑕᐅᔪᑦ ᑲᔪᕐᓂᑦ.

The tiny blossoms of kallait kallaqutillu appear briefly in the very early summer. In this picture, the new season's green leaves are crowded amongst the brown leaves of the previous season.

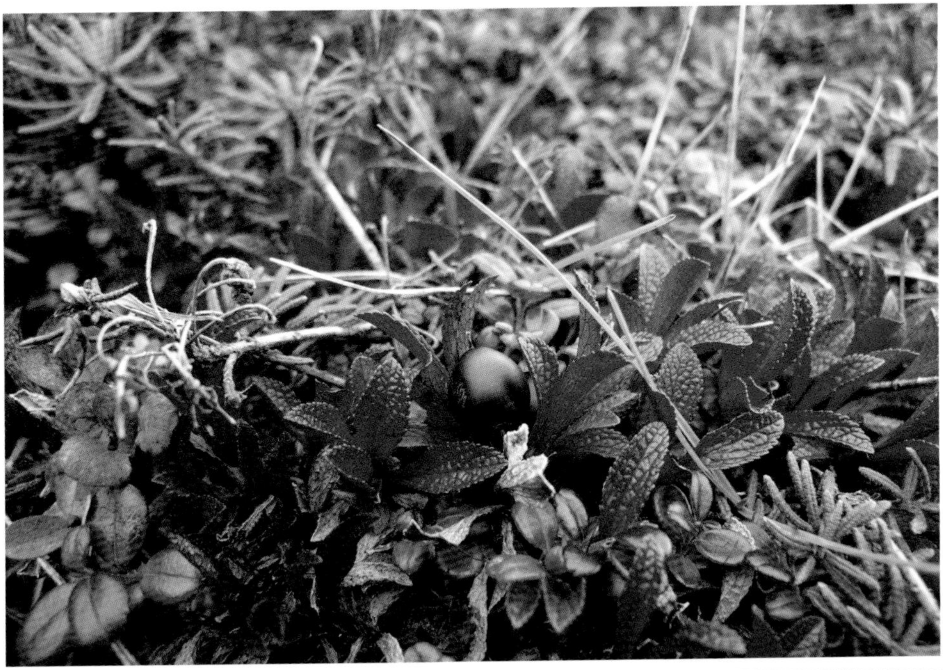

ᑲᓪᓚᐃᑦ ᑲᓪᓚᖁᑎᓪᓗ ᐱᕈᖅᐸᓪᓕᐊᔪᑦ ᓂᒐᕕᓯᒪᓪᓗᑎᑦ ᐃᕕᖕᓄᑦ, ᐊᓯᖏᓐᓄᓪᓗ ᐸᐅᖕᒐᓄᑦ, ᐊᒻᒪᓗ ᖁᔪᒃᑖᖅᐸᓄᑦ (ᑏᖕᒎᐊᒃᓴᐃᑦ). ᐅᑭᐊᒃᓴᓕᖅᑎᓪᓗᒍ, ᐊᔾᔨᒌᖕᒋᑦᑐᑦ ᑲᓪᓚᐃᑦ ᐋᓚᓯᐅᑉ ᐃᓪᓗᖓᑕ ᓯᓚᑖᓂᑦ ᖁᕐᓂᖅᓯᖅᑲᑕᖅᑐᑦ ᐱᕈᓈᕐᖓᒪᑕ. ᑲᓪᓚᖁᑎᓪᓕ (ᐅᖅᑲᐅᔾᔨᖕᒋᑦ) ᐊᐅᐸᓪᓚᓐᓇᑦᑐᑰᓘᓕᖅᐸᑦᑐᑎᒃ.

This photo shows kallait kallaqutillu growing in a tangle with grasses, cranberries, and *qijuktaaqpait* (Labrador tea; p. 81). In the early fall, the kallait that grows around Aalasi's house turns black as it ripens. The kallaqutit turn a blazing red.

ᑕᕐᑲᓂᐊᓘᔮᕐᑐᑎᒃ. ᐊᐅᐸᓪᓚᓇᒃᓯᕐᑲᑦᑕᕐᑐᑦ ᐅᑭᐊᒃᓵᒃᑯᑦ. ᐱᕈᕐᓯᐊᖑᓕᑦ ᖁᕐᓱᕈᕝᑐᑎᑦ ᓯᕙᓂᕈᑎᖕᖑᐊᑯᓘᔮᕐᑲᑦᑕᕐᑐᑦ. ᑲᓪᓚᐃᓪᓂ ᐊᒻᒪᓗᑭᓵᓪᓚᓇᐅᕙᑦᑐᑦ. ᕿᑭᕐᑕᓂ ᓇᓂᔭᐅᓲᑦ ᕿᕐᓂᕐᑑᕙᑦᑐᑦ ᐱᕈᓅᕐᓯᒪᓂᕐᑐᑎᒃ, ᑭᕙᓪᓕᕐᒥᓂ ᓇᓂᔭᐅᕐᑲᑦᑕᕐᑐᑦ ᐊᐅᐸᕐᓯᖕᒑᕐᑲᑦᑕᕐᑐᑦ ᐱᕈᓅᕐᓯᒪᓂᕐᑎᓪᓗᒋᑦ. ᑕᒪᕐᒦᓪᓂ ᓇᓂᔭᐅᓲᖑᕗᑦ ᕿᑎᕐᒥᐅᓂ.

Kallait kallaqutillu is common in the southern Qikiqtani, some parts of the Kivalliq, and in many parts of the Kitikmeot. Kallait kallaqutillu can be distinguished from *kigutangirnait naqutillu* (blueberry; p. 75) by the slightly jagged edges of its leaves (kigutangirnait naqutillu has smooth-edged leaves). The leaves are small with easily visible veins. They turn bright red in the fall. The flowers are pale yellow green and shaped like tiny bells. The kallait are round and smooth. The ones that are commonly found in the southern Qikiqtani are usually black when ripe, while the ones found in some parts of the Kivalliq are red when ripe. Both types are found in the Kitikmeot.

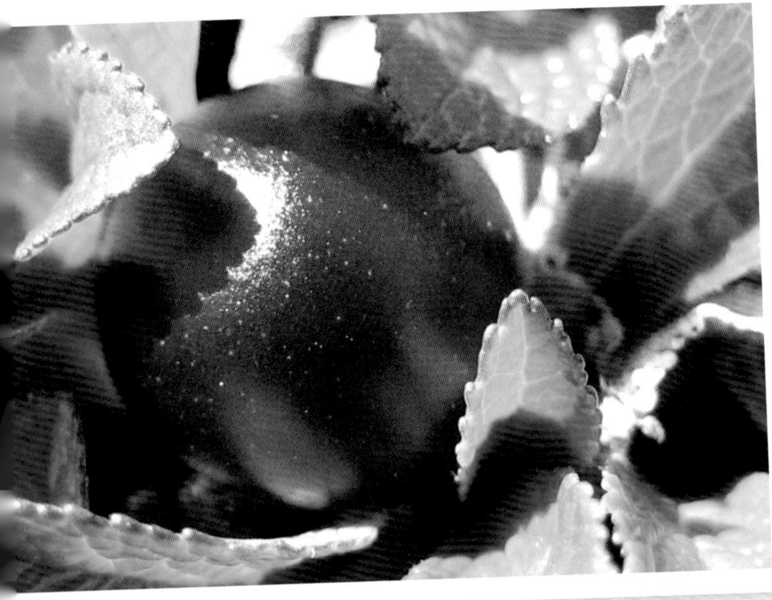

ᐊᐅᔭᐅᑉ ᕿᑎᕐᐸᓯᐊᓂ ᐃᕐᑲᓗᐃᑦ ᓯᓚᑎᑦᑎᐊᖕᒐᓂ, ᑲᓪᓚᐃᑦ (ᐸᐅᕐᖕᒐᖕᒋᑦ) ᐊᐅᐸᕐᑐᐃᑦ ᐱᕈᓅᓚᐅᕐᑎᓐᓇᒋᑦ ᐊᒻᒪᓗ ᑲᓪᓚᕐᑯᑎᑦ (ᐅᕐᑲᐅᔭᖕᒋᑦ) ᑐᖕᒍᑦᑐᓇᑦᑐᑎᒃ.

Mid-season near Iqaluit, the kallait are red before they ripen and the kallaqutit are bright green.

ᑭᒍᑕᖏᕐᓇᐃᑦ ᓇᖁᑎᓪᓗ
Kigutangirnait Naqutillu / Blueberry

ᐃᓄᒃᑎᑐᑦ, ᑭᒍᑕᖏᕐᓇᐃᑦ (ᐊᑕᐅᓯᐅᓪᓗᓂ: ᑭᒍᑕᖏᕐᓇᖅ) ᐊᒻᒪ ᓇᖁᑎᑦ ᐅᖃᐅᓯᖃᖅᑐᑦ ᐅᖃᐅᓴᖏᓐᓂᑦ. ᑕᕝᕙᓂᓕ ᑕᐃᑲᑕᓐᓂᐊᖅᑕᕗᑦ ᑭᒍᑕᖏᕐᓇᑦ ᓇᖁᑎᓪᓗ"). ᑭᒍᑕᖏᕐᓇᐃᑦ, ᑐᑭᖃᖅᑐᖅ "ᑭᒍᑕᐃᕆᑏᑦ" ᐊᑎᖅᑲᐅᑎᒋᒻᒪᒋᑦ ᑭᒍᑎᐅᑉ ᓱᕿᓐᓂᖏᑦ ᑐᖑᔪᖅᑰᓕᖅᑲᑦᑕᖅᒪᑕ ᐲᓚᐅᙱᓯᖕᒐᖅᑎᓪᓗᒋᑦ.

In Inuktitut, *kigutangirnait* (singular: *kigutangirnaq*) refers to the berries of the plant and *naqutit* refers to the leaves of the plant. Here, we refer to the plant generally as *kigutangirnat naqutillu* ("kigutangirnat and naqutit"). Kigutangirnait, which means "that which causes the teeth to be removed," are named for what it looks like when dark blue pieces remain on the teeth.

ᑭᒍᑕᖏᕐᓇᐃᑦ ᓇᖁᑎᓪᓗ ᓄᓂᕗᑦᑕᐅᔭᒪᓂᖅᐹᖑᕕᑦᓚᐃᔭᑦ. ᓄᓇᕗᒻᒥ ᐱᑕᖅᑲᔭᒻᒪᑕ. ᑖᒃᑯᐊ ᐊᔾᔨᖏᑦᓚᕆᒻᒪᒋᑦ ᐸᐅᖕᖓᐃᑦ ᐸᐅᖕᖓᖁᑎᓪᓗ ᐅᖃᐅᔾᔨᖏᑕ ᑭᓪᓕᖏᑦ ᑐᑭᓕᐊᑦᑎᐊᖅᒪᑕ

ᐅᑯᐊ ᑭᒍᑕᖏᕐᓇᐃᑦ ᓂᕿᑐᐃᓐᓇᕿᐊᖅᑲᓕᖅᑐᖅ! ᑭᖕᒍᑕᖏᕐᓇᕐᓂᒃ ᓄᓂᕙᖕᓂᖅ ᑲᔪᖏᑦᑎᐊᕆᐊᖃᖅᐳᖅ ᑕᑉᐱᑦᑐᓂᓗ. ᑖᒃᑯᐊ ᓂᕐᒪ ᓱᓚᒃᓴᐃᑦ ᐃᔾᔭᖅᓯᒪᒡᒍᔪᑦ ᓇᖁᑏᑦ ᐊᑎᖏᓐᓂᒃ.

These kigutangirnait are ready to eat! Collecting kigutangirnait requires dedication and a keen eye. The tiny treats are often hidden beneath their naqutit.

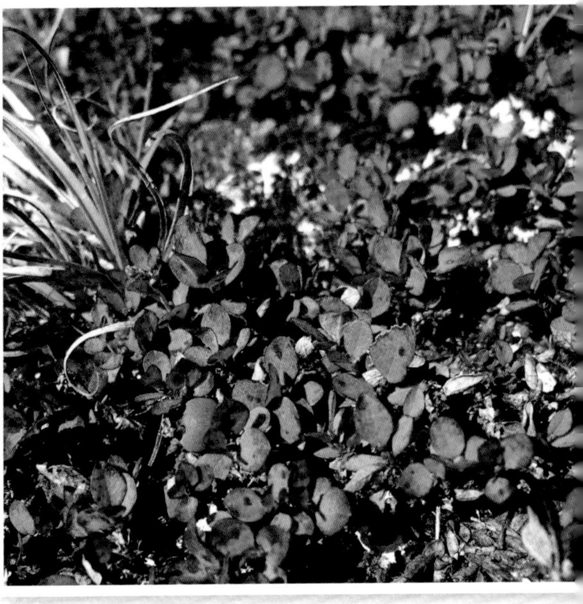

(ᐸᐅᖓᐃᑦ ᐸᐅᖓᖁᑎᓪᓗ ᑲᐱᓪᓛᓇᖅᑐᑯᓘᒻᒪᑕ). ᐊᐅᔭᒃᑯᑦ ᐅᖃᐅᔭᖏᑦ ᑐᖑᑦᑐᓇᑦᑐᑎᒃ ᐊᐅᐸᓪᓚᓇᓕᖃᑦᑕᖅᑐᑦ ᐅᑭᐊᒃᓵᖓ. ᓇᑲᖏᑦ ᑕᑭᓪᓕᒻᒪᓇᖃᑦᑕᖅᑐᑦ, ᑭᓯᐊᓂ 15 ᓯᐊᓐᑎᒦᑐᒥᑦ ᑕᑭᓂᖅᓴᐅᓕᕈᓐᓇᕐᑎᑦ. ᐱᕈᖅᓯᐊᖏᓪᓚ ᖃᑯᖅᑕᐅᖃᑦᑕᖅᑐᑦ ᐊᐅᐸᕈᔪᒃᑐᑎᓪᓗ, ᓯᕙᓂᕈᑎᕐᓛᙳᐊᑯᓘᔭᑐᑎᒃ. ᑭᒍᑕᖏᕐᓇᐃᑦ ᑐᖑᔪᖅᑑᖃᑦᑕᖅᑐᑦ ᐱᕈᓃᖅᓯᒪᓕᖅᑐᑎᒃ. ᐱᕈᓕᓵᖅᑎᓪᓗᒋᓪᓕ ᖃᑯᖅᑕᐸᔫᕙᑦᑐᑎᒃ.

Kigutangirnait naqutillu is perhaps the most sought-after berry plant. It is common in most parts of Nunavut. This plant is easily distinguishable from *kallait kallaqutillu* (bearberry; p. 75) by the smooth edges of its leaves (kallait kallaqutillu has slightly jagged edges). The leaves are bluish green in summer and turn bright red in autumn. The stems can grow quite long but are usually less than 15 cm tall. The flowers are pink and white, shaped like tiny bells. Kigutangirnait are round and blue when ripe. Before they are ripe, they are almost white.

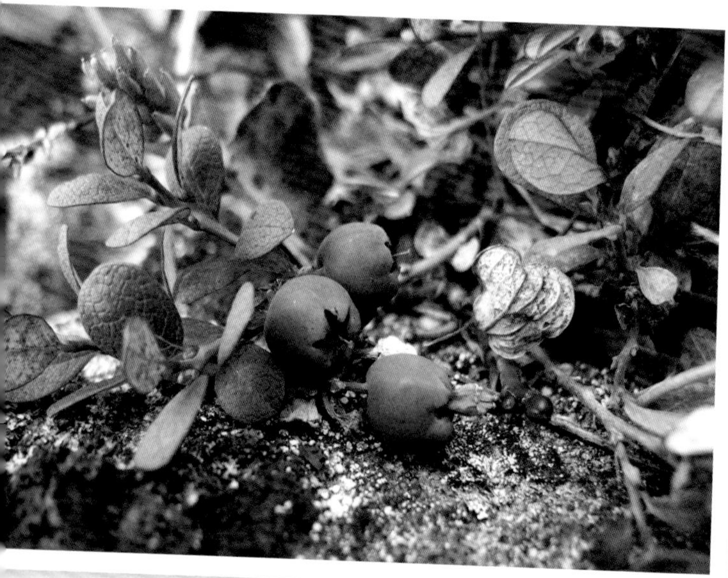

ᓇᖁᑏᑦ ᐅᖃᐅᔭᖏᑦ ᐊᐅᐸᖅᓯᓲᑦ ᐅᑭᐊᒃᓵᒃᑯᑦ.

The leaves of kigutangirnait turn red in the fall.

ᑭᒍᑕᖏᕐᓇᖁᑎᑦ ᓄᕗᕈᑎᖏᑦ ᕿᓚᒥᑯᓗᒃ
ᐊᐅᔭᒃᑯᑦ ᓴᖅᑮᔭᑲᐃᓐᓇᓲᑦ. ᖃᑯᖅᑕᐅᔪᑦ
ᐊᐅᐸᕈᔪᓐᓂᐊᕐᔪᖃᖅᑐᑎᒃ.

The tiny blossoms of kigutangirnait naqutillu appear very briefly at the beginning of summer. They are white with delicate blushes of pink.

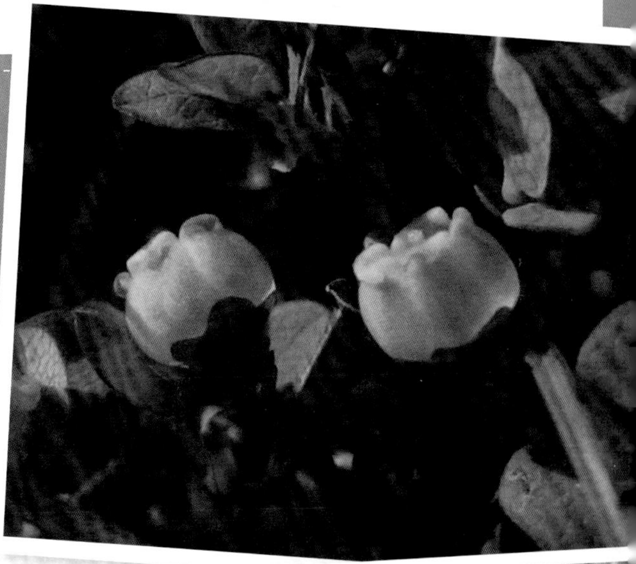

ᓇᖁᑎᑦ (ᐅᖃᐅᔭᖏᑦ) ᑭᓪᓕᖏᑦ ᒪᓂᕿᑦᑐᑦ,
ᑲᓪᓚᖁᑎᓪᓕ (ᐅᖃᐅᔭᖏᑦ) ᑭᓪᓕᖏᑦ ᒪᓂᕿᓐᓇᑎᒃ.
ᑖᓐᓇ ᐅᖃᐅᔭᖅ ᓴᐅᒥᓐᓃᑦᑐᑦ ᑎᓗᖅᑯᖓᓂᑦ
ᑕᑯᔅᓴᐅᔪᖅ ᑲᓪᓚᖁᑎᐅᔪᖅ (ᐅᖃᐅᔭᖏᑦ),
ᐊᓯᖏᓪᓕ ᐅᖃᐅᔭᐃᑦ ᑕᑯᔅᓴᐅᔪᑦ ᓇᖁᑎᐅᔪᑦ
(ᑭᒍᑕᖏᕐᓇᐃᑦ ᐅᖃᐅᔭᖏᑦ).

Naqutit have smooth edges, while kallaqutit (bearberry leaves) have bumpy edges. The leaf at the bottom left-hand corner of this picture is kallaqutit, while the other leaves in this picture are naqutit.

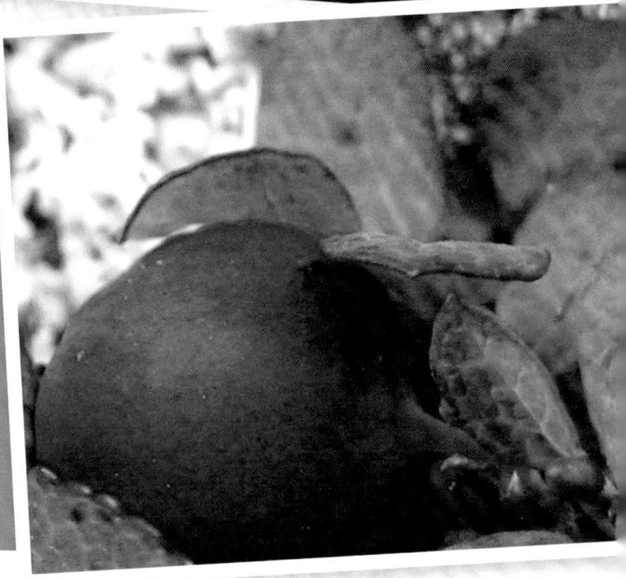

ᐸᐅᕐᖓᓂᑦ ᐊᑐᕐᓂᐊᕐᓗᓂ

Using Berry Plants

ᐸᐅᕐᖓᐃᑦ ᐊᔾᔨᒌᖕᒋᑦᑐᑦ ᐳᑯᑐᐃᓐᓇᖅᓴᐃᓐᓇᐃᑦ. ᑭᒍᑕᖕᒋᕐᓇᐃᑦ ᓲᕐᓇᓛᖑᓪᓗᑎᒃ, ᑭᓯᐊᓂ ᐸᐅᕐᖓᐃᑦ ᐊᒻᒪ ᑲᓪᓚᐃᑦ ᒪᒪᖅᑐᑯᓗᐃᑦ ᓂᕿᑦᑎᐊᕙᐅᓪᓗᑎᓪᓗ. ᐸᐅᕐᖓᐃᑦ ᑕᒪᒃᑯᐊᑦ ᖃᖓᑐᐃᓐᓇᒃᑯᑦ ᓂᕆᔭᒃᓴᐅᓲᖑᔪᑦ—ᐱᕈᓕᓵᖅᑎᓪᓗᒋᑦ ᐅᕙᓘᓐᓃᑦ ᐱᕈᓈᖅᓯᒪᓕᖅᑎᓪᓗᒋᑦ. ᑭᒍᑕᖕᒋᕐᓇᐃᑦ ᐸᐅᕐᖓᐃᓪᓗ ᐱᕈᓈᖅᓯᒪᓕᖅᑎᓪᓗᒋᑦ ᒪᒪᓛᖑᔪᑦ. (ᐅᑭᐊᒃᓴᓕᖃᑖᖅᑎᓪᓗᒍ), ᑭᓯᐊᓂᓕ ᐱᕈᓈᓚᐅᖅᑎᓐᓇᒋᑦ ᑲᓪᓚᐃᑦ ᒪᒪᕐᓂᖅᐹᖑᖅᑲᑦᑕᖅᐳᑦ.

The berries of all three plants can be eaten fresh from the plant. *Kigutangirnait* (blueberries; p. 75) are the sweetest, but *paurngait* (crowberries; p. 68) and *kallait* (bearberries; p. 72) are also enjoyable and nutritious. All three types of berries can be eaten at any time—ripe or unripe. Kigutangirnait and paurngait taste best when they are ripe (in the early fall), but kallait are most delicious before they are ripe.

ᐱᓂᖅᓴᐅᔪᖅ ᓂᕆᓗᐊᑲᐅᑎᒋᖕᒋᒃᑯᕕᑦ ᐸᐅᕐᖓᓂᑦ. ᐸᐅᕐᖓᐃᑦ ᐱᓗᐊᕐᓗᒋᑦ ᓈᙳᓕᕐᓇᕐᒪᑕ. ᓂᕆᔭᒃᓴᑑᔭᕆᐊᖅᑲᖕᒋᒃᑭᕗᑦ ᑳᓗᐊᖅᑐᒧᑦ ᓂᕆᑦᑎᐊᖅᑲᑦᑕᖅᓯᒪᖕᒋᑦᑐᒧᑦ. ᑭᓯᐊᓂᓕᑦᑕᐅ, ᑭᒍᑕᖕᒋᕐᓇᐃᑦ ᑲᓪᓚᐃᓪᓗ ᐃᓱᒪᐃᓐᓇᖅ ᓂᕆᕐᑯᔦᑦ.

It is best to avoid eating too many paurngait all at once. Eating too many paurngait may cause a stomach ache. Also, paurngait should not be relied on when a person is very hungry or malnourished. However, it is safe to eat as many kigutangirnait and kallait as you wish.

ᐸᐅᕐᖓᐃᑦ ᑭᒍᑕᖕᒋᕐᓇᐃᓪᓗ ᓂᕆᓂᐊᖅᑕᓐᓄᑦ ᐃᓚᓕᐅᑎᔪᓐᓇᖅᑎᐊᖅᑕᐃᑦ. ᐅᖅᑲᓖᒪᕐᒥᑦ ᐊᑯᓕᐅᕈᑎᑦ ᒪᓕᓪᓗᒋᑦ ᓇᓕᐊᓐᓂᑐᐃᓐᓇᖅ ᐃᓚᓕᐅᑎᔪᓐᓇᖅᑖᒃᑭᑦ. ᓂᕿᓕᐅᕈᑎᓂᑦ ᐅᖅᑲᓖᒪᕐᒥᑦ ᐱᑕᖅᑲᕐᒥᒻᒪᑦ ᐃᖅᑲᓗᓕᐅᕈᑎᑦ, ᐸᐅᕐᖓᖅᑲᖅᑐᕐᒥᑦ, ᐊᒻᒪᓗ ᑲᑎᖅᓱᖅᓯᒪᔦᑦ ᐱᕈᖅᑐᕕᓂᑦ ᑐᖅᑕᐃᑦ (ᑐᖅᑕᐃᑦ, ᓇᑲᖕᒪᑕ ᐃᓚᖕᒪ; p. 63). ᑭᒍᑕᖕᒋᕐᓇᐃᑦ ᐸᐅᕐᖓᐃᓪᓗ ᐸᓚᐅᓖᓕᐊᒧᑦ ᐃᓚᓕᐅᔾᔭᐅᔪᓐᓇᖅᑐᑦ. ᑭᓯᐊᓂ ᐸᐅᕐᖓᓂᑦ ᐸᓚᐅᓖᓕᐊᑦ ᐃᓚᓪᓗᒋᑦ ᐱᐅᓂᖅᓴᐃᑦ ᑭᒍᑕᖕᒋᕐᓇᐃᑦ ᐅᐊᑦᑎᐊᕈᕐᓇᓵᕈᒥᓇᕐᒪᑕ. ᐅᓪᓗᒥᐅᓕᖅᑐᕐᑕ ᐸᐅᕐᖓᐃᑦ ᑭᒍᑕᖕᒋᕐᓇᐃᓪᓗ ᔹᒻᓕᐊᖑᕙᓕᖅᑐᑦ ᐊᒻᒪᓗ ᓲᕐᓇᖅᑐᓕᐊᖑᕙᓕᖅᑐᑎᑦ.

Paurngait and kigutangirnait can be made into many different dishes, such as *aluit* (puddings). There is also a recipe for a salad of char, paurngait, and *tuqtait* (alpine bistort rhizomes; p. 63). Kigutangirnait and paurngait can be added to bannock. But Aalasi suggests that it may be best to use paurngait in bannock because fresh kigutangirnait are such a precious treat. These days, people also use kigutangirnait and paurngait in jams, jellies, and desserts.

ᐋᓚᓯ ᐃᖅᑲᐅᒪᔪᖅ ᐃᓚᕇᓂᒫᑦᑎᐊᑦ ᐸᐅᖕᖓᓂᑦ ᑭᒍᑕᖏᕐᓇᓂᓪᓗ ᓄᓂᕙᖅᑲᑦᑕᓚᐅᖅᓯᒪᒐᒥ ᐊᐅᔭᐅᓂᖀᖕᒐᑦ. ᐊᒡᒐᓐᓄᑦ ᓄᓂᕙᒐᔅᓴᐅᔪᑦ, ᐅᓪᓗᒥᐅᓕᖅᑐᖅᑕ ᑭᓯᐊᓂ ᓄᓂᕙᐅᑎᖅᑲᖅᑲᑦᑕᓕᖅᒥᔪᑦ. ᓄᓂᕙᐅᑎᐅᑉ ᐊᑯᓂᖕᒋᑎᒍ ᐸᐅᖕᒐᑦ ᐲᑦᑎᐊᖅᑲᑦᑕᖅᑐᑦ ᓇᑲᖕᒋᓐᓂᑦ.

Aalasi recalls that her entire family would work together to collect kigutangirnait and paurngait in the summer. The berries can be hand-picked, but some people prefer to use a rake-like tool called a *nunivauti*. The fingers of a nunivauti pull the berries off the stems all at once.

ᑲᓪᓚᖁᑏᑦ, ᑲᓪᓚᐃᑦ ᐱᕈᖅᕕᖕᒋᑦ, ᒪᒪᖅᑐᒥᒃ, ᑏᓕᐊᕆᔭᒃᓴᐅᕗᑦ (ᐸᐅᖕᒐᐃᑦ ᐊᓯᖕᒋᑦ ᐅᖅᑲᐅᔭᖕᒋᑦ ᑏᑦᑎᐊᕆᓂᐊᓂᔭᒃᓴᐅᖕᒋᒻᒪᑕ). ᐅᖅᑲᐅᔭᖕᒋᑦ ᓇᑲᖕᒋᓪᓗ ᖃᖕᒪᑐᐃᓐᓇᒃᑯᑦ ᓄᐊᑕᒃᓴᐅᕗᑦ, ᑐᖑᔪᖅᑕᐅᑎᓪᓗᒋᑦ ᑲᔫᑎᓪᓗᒋᓘᓐᓃᑦ. ᑲᓪᓚᖁᑎᓂᑦ ᑏᓕᐅᕐᓂᐊᕈᕕᑦ, ᑎᒍᒥᐊᕋᒃᓴᓪᓗᐊᓂᑦ ᓇᑲᓂᑦ ᐅᖅᑲᐅᔭᖅᑲᖅᓗᒋᑦ ᑎᖅᑎᑎᑦᑎᓗᑎᑦ ᐊᑯᓂᐊᓗᒃ. ᑲᓪᓚᖁᑎᓂᑦ ᑏᓕᐊᕆᓯᒪᔪᑦ ᐋᓚᓯᐅᑉ ᒪᒪᕆᓛᑦᑎᐊᕆᕙ.

Kallaqutiit, the leaves of bearberry, make a tangy, delicious tea (the leaves of the other two berry plants are not good for tea). The leaves and stems can be collected at any time, green or brown. To make kallaqutiit tea, boil a handful of stems with leaves for a long time. Kallaqutiit tea is Aalasi's favourite tea.

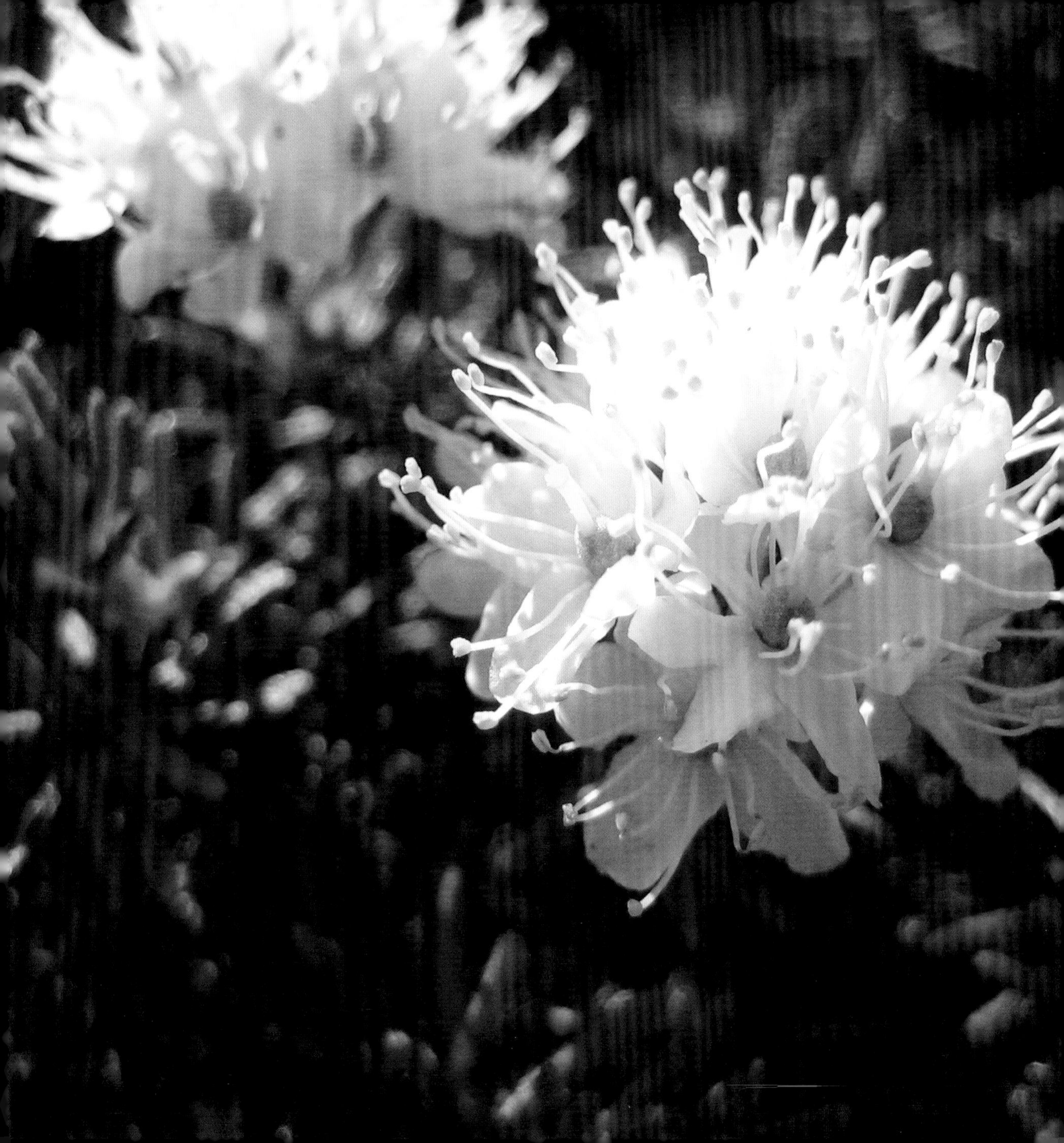

ᕿᔪᒃᑖᖅᐸᐃᑦ

Qijuktaaqpait / Labrador Tea

ᐊᐅᔭᒃᑯᑦ ᕿᔪᑦᑖᖅᐸᐃᑦ ᐱᕈᓕᕐᖅᑎᓪᓗᒋᑦ ᖃᒃᑰᓪᓗᑎᒃ ᐅᓪᓗᓇᐊᑯᓘᔮᖅᑕᑕᖅᑐᑦ ᓄᓇᔾᒥᑦ. ᓇᓗᓇᖏᑦᑐᑯᓘᓯᑦ ᑖᓪᓕᒪᓂᓪᓗ ᐱᕈᖅᑐᖅᑲᖅᑐᑎᒃ. ᐅᖃᐅᔭᖏᑦ ᑐᖑᑦᑐᓇᑦᑐᑎᒃ ᐊᒥᑦᑐᑯᑖᖑᔪᑦ ᐊᑖᓅᓇᐊᖕᒐᖅᑰᕕᓪᓗᑎᒃ, ᒥᖅᑯᑎᙳᐊᑯᓘᔮᖅᑐᑦ. ᐊᑎᖏᑦ ᑲᔪᕈᔪᐃᑦ ᐊᐅᐸᕈᔪᑦᑐᑎᒃ ᒥᖅᑯᖃᖅᑐᑎᓪᓗ. ᐱᕈᕝᕕᖏᑦ 15 ᓰᓐᑎᒦᑐᓂᒃ ᑕᑭᓂᖃᖅᑕᑕᖅᑐᑦ.

In early summer, the blossoms of *qijuktaaqpait* (Labrador tea) look like bright white stars on the tundra. They have five white petals and grow in distinct clusters. The dark green leaves are narrow and the edges roll under, making them look like needles. Their undersides are covered with rust-coloured hairs. The stems grow in mats and are usually no longer than 15 cm.

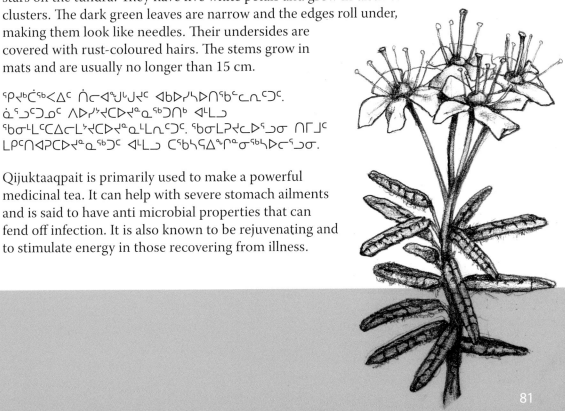

ᕿᔪᒃᑖᖅᐸᐃᑦ ᑏᓕᐊᖑᒡᒍᔪᑦ ᐊᑲᐅᓯᔅᐅᑎᖃᑦᑕᓇᑦᑐᑦ. ᓈᕐᓗᑦᑐᓄᑦ ᐱᐅᓯᔾᔪᑕᐅᔪᓐᓇᖅᑐᑎᒃ ᐊᒻᒪᓗ ᖃᓂᒪᑦᑕᐃᓕᒪᔾᔪᑕᐅᔪᓐᓇᒻᒪᑎᑦᑐᑦ. ᖃᓂᒪᕈᔪᓚᐅᕐᓗᓂ ᑎᒥᒧᑦ ᒪᑭᑦᑎᐊᕈᑕᐅᔪᓐᓇᖅᑐᑦ ᐊᒻᒪᓗ ᑕᕐᖃᓯᕐᐃᖏᓐᓂᖅᓴᐅᓕᕐᓗᓂ.

Qijuktaaqpait is primarily used to make a powerful medicinal tea. It can help with severe stomach ailments and is said to have anti microbial properties that can fend off infection. It is also known to be rejuvenating and to stimulate energy in those recovering from illness.

ᐱᔾᔪᑎᒋᓪᓗᒍ ᑭᓱᐊᓂ, ᓴᙱᓂᐊᓗᐊ, ᕿᔪᑦᑖᖅᐸᐃᑦ ᐊᔾᔨᖐᖕᒋᑦᑐᑦ ᐃᒻᒥᒃᑯᑦ ᑏᓕᐊᖕᒍᖅᑲᑦᑕᖕᒋᑦᑐᑦ ᐊᑲᐅᓯᓴᐅᑕᐅᓂᐊᕋᓗᐊᕈᓂ. ᑏᓕᐊᓇᓂᐊᕈᕕᐅᓪᓚ ᐃᓚᓕᐅᔾᔩᖕᒎᕐᔭᖅᑐᑎᑦ ᕿᔪᑦᑖᖅᐸᒥᑦ ᑏᓕᐊᓇᔭᓃᖅᓯᒪᔪᒧᑦ ᐸᐅᓐᓇᒻᒥᑦ, ᐊᑕᐅᓯᑯᑖᒥᒃ ᑏᓕᐊᓇᔭᐃᑦ ᐃᓗᐃᓐᓇᕐᓗ (ᐸᐅᓐᓇᐃᑦ; p. 47) ᐊᓯᖕᒋᓐᓄᑦ ᓅᓐᓃᑦ ᐅᕝᕙᓅᓐᓃᑦ ᓂᐅᕕᕐᕕᒻᒦᙳᖅᑐᒥᑦ ᑏᒥᑦ. ᑏᓕᐊᓐᓄᑦ ᐆᑐᐃᓐᓇᕿᓐᓇᖅᑕᐃᑦ ᐅᕝᕙᓅᓐᓂᑦ ᑯᕕᔭᓃᖅᓯᒪᔭᓐᓄᑦ ᐃᖖᒍᓯᕐᒧᑦ ᑏᒧᑦ.

However, because of its potency, the Arctic variety of qijuktaaqpait should not be used to make medicinal tea on its own. To make a medicinal tea from qijuktaaqpait, add a single sprig of qijuktaaqpait to any other tea, such as *paunnait* (dwarf fireweed; p. 47) and other land teas, or even store-bought teas. The sprig can be added for a few minutes to the teapot, or right into the cup.

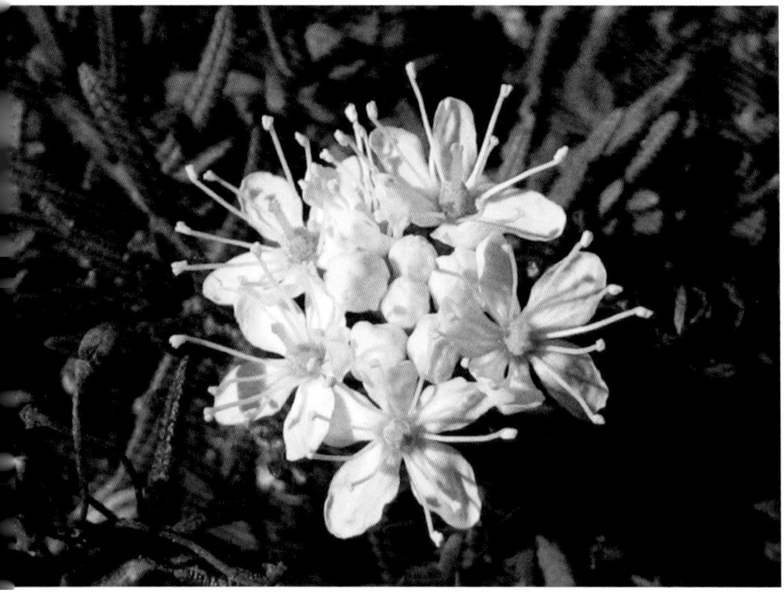

ᕿᔪᒃᑖᖅᐸᐃᑦ ᑏᓕᐊᓇᓂᐊᕐᓗᒍ ᒪᒪᕐᓂᖅᐹᖑᔪᖅ ᓴᙱᓂᖅᐹᖑᓪᓗᑎᓪᓗ ᑎᒥᒥᑦ ᐊᑲᐅᓯᓴᐅᑎᑦ ᓄᐊᑕᐅᒍᑎᒃ ᐅᑭᐊᒃᓵᒥᑦ. ᖁᐊᖅᑎᓯᒪᓱᖕᒐᕐᓗᒍ ᐊᕐᖄᒍᓕᒫᕐᒧᑦ ᐃᓕᒃᑯᐊᓇᔭᒃᓴᐅᔪᑦ ᓴᙱᓂᖅᑲᑦᑎᐊᖏᓐᓇᕐᓂᐊᕐᒪᑦ.

ᐊᐅᔭᓖᒃᑯᑦ ᕿᔪᒃᑖᖅᐸᐃᑦ ᐅᑦᓗᓇᐊᑯᓘᔮᖅᑐᖅ.

The starry blossoms of qijuktaaqpait are shown here in early summer.

Qijuktaaqpait makes the most delicious and medicinally powerful tea if it is collected in the fall. It can be used all year long if it is kept frozen to preserve its strength.

ᕐᑭᔪᒃᑖᕐᒃᐸᐃᑦ ᑭᑦᑕᒧᑦ ᓴᓗᒻᒪᕐᒃᓴᐃᔾᔭᑕᐅᔭᓐᓇᕆᕗᑦ. ᓴᓗᒻᒪᕐᒃᓴᐃᔾᔭᑎᒥᓂᐊᕐᓗᒍ, ᑎᕐᒃᑎᑦᑐᒦᑎᑲᐃᓐᓇᕐᓗᒋᑦ ᑎᒍᑦᓗᐊᕐᒃᓴᐃᑦ. ᐃᒪᕐᒃ ᑎᓴᐃᕐᔩᒥᑉᐸᑦ ᕐᑲᑦᓗᓈᕐᒃᑕᒥᑦ ᒪᓴᑦᑎᓇᓗᑎᑦ ᕐᑲᔪᖓᓂ ᑖᓐᓇ ᑭᑦᑕᕐᒥᑦ ᓴᓗᒻᒪᕐᒃᓴᐃᔾᔭᑎᒥᑕᕐᓗᒍ. ᕐᑭᔪᒃᑖᕐᒃᐸᐃᑦ ᐊᑲᐅᓯᓴᐅᑎᖕᒥᑦ ᑭᑦᑕᕐᒥᑦ ᓱᑯᖖᒋᑎᑦᑎᔭᓐᓇᕐᒪᑦ.

Qijuktaaqpait can also be used to clean wounds. To use it as a cleanser, boil a handful in a pot of water. When the water has cooled enough, soak a cloth in it and use the cloth to clean the wound. The antimicrobial properties of qijuktaaqpait will decrease the risk of infection.

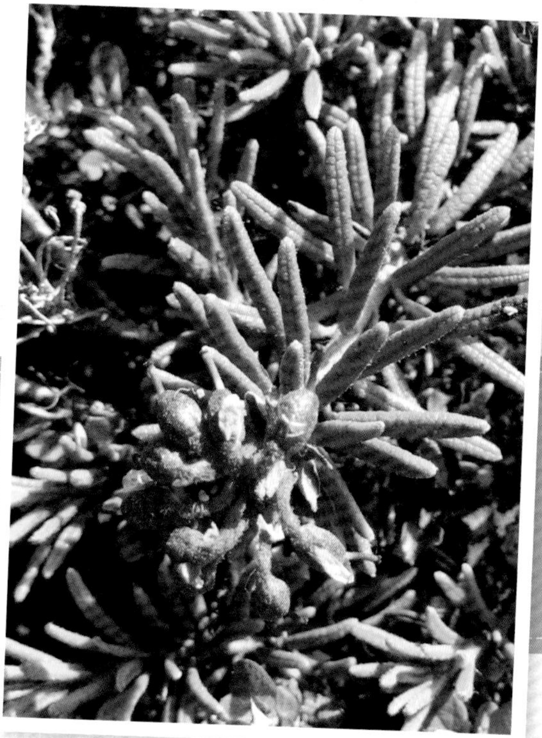

ᐊᒥᓱᓄᑦ ᕐᑭᔪᒃᑖᕐᒃᐸᐃᑦ ᑎᐱᖓ ᒪᒪᕆᔭᐅᒻᒪᑦ. ᐃᑦᓗᓐᓄᑦ ᓇᒧᐃᓐᓇᕐᒃ ᐃᓕᐅᕐᒃᑲᕈᓐᓇᕐᒥᔭᐃᑦ ᑎᐱᑦᑎᐊᓂᒍᑕᐅᓂᐊᕐᒪᑦ. ᑎᐱᕐᒃᑦᑎᐊᕈᓐᓇᕐᓂᕐᒃᐹᖑᔪᕐᒃ ᐃᒻᒫᕐᔪᔅᓯᒪᓗᒋᑦ ᐸᓂᕐᒃᑎᑦᑕᐃᓕᒪᓗᒋᑦ.

Many people find the spicy scent of qijuktaaqpait to be soothing. It can be placed throughout the home to be enjoyed. It will smell best if it is set in a small amount of water to keep it moist.

ᐊᐅᔭᐅᔅᓴᓕᕐᒃᑎᑦᓗᒍ ᕐᑭᔪᒃᑖᕐᒃᐸᐃᑦ. ᐅᑦᓗᓇᐊᖕᒍᔮᓚᐅᕐᒃᑐᕐᒃ ᐱᑕᕐᒃᑯᓐᓃᕋᓗᐊᕐᒃᑎᓗᒋᑦ ᑭᓯᐊᓂ ᐅᕐᒃᑲᐅᔭᖕᒋᓐᓄᑦ ᓱᓕ ᓇᓂᔭᓐᓇᕋᔭᕐᒃᑕᐃᑦ.

By late summer, qijuktaaqpait's starry white blossoms have gone, but you can still find this plant by its distinctive leaves.

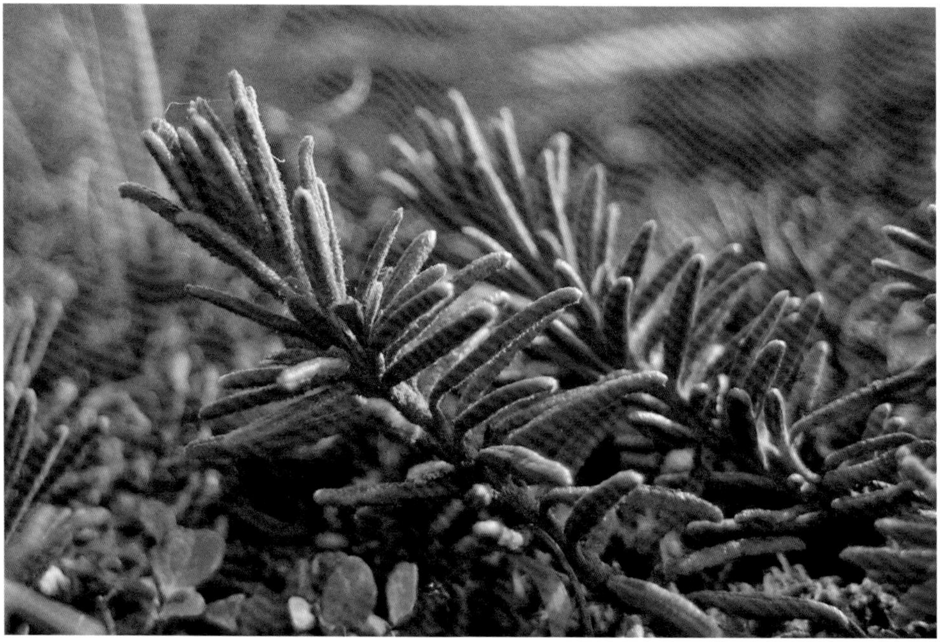

ᕿᔪᒃᑖᖅᐸᐃᑦ ᓴᙱᓂᖅᐹᖑᔪᑦ ᒪᒪᕐᓂᖅᐹᖑᓪᓗᑎᓪᓗ ᐅᑭᐊᒃᓵᒃᑯᑦ.

Qijuktaaqpait is most delicious and medicinally powerful in the early fall.

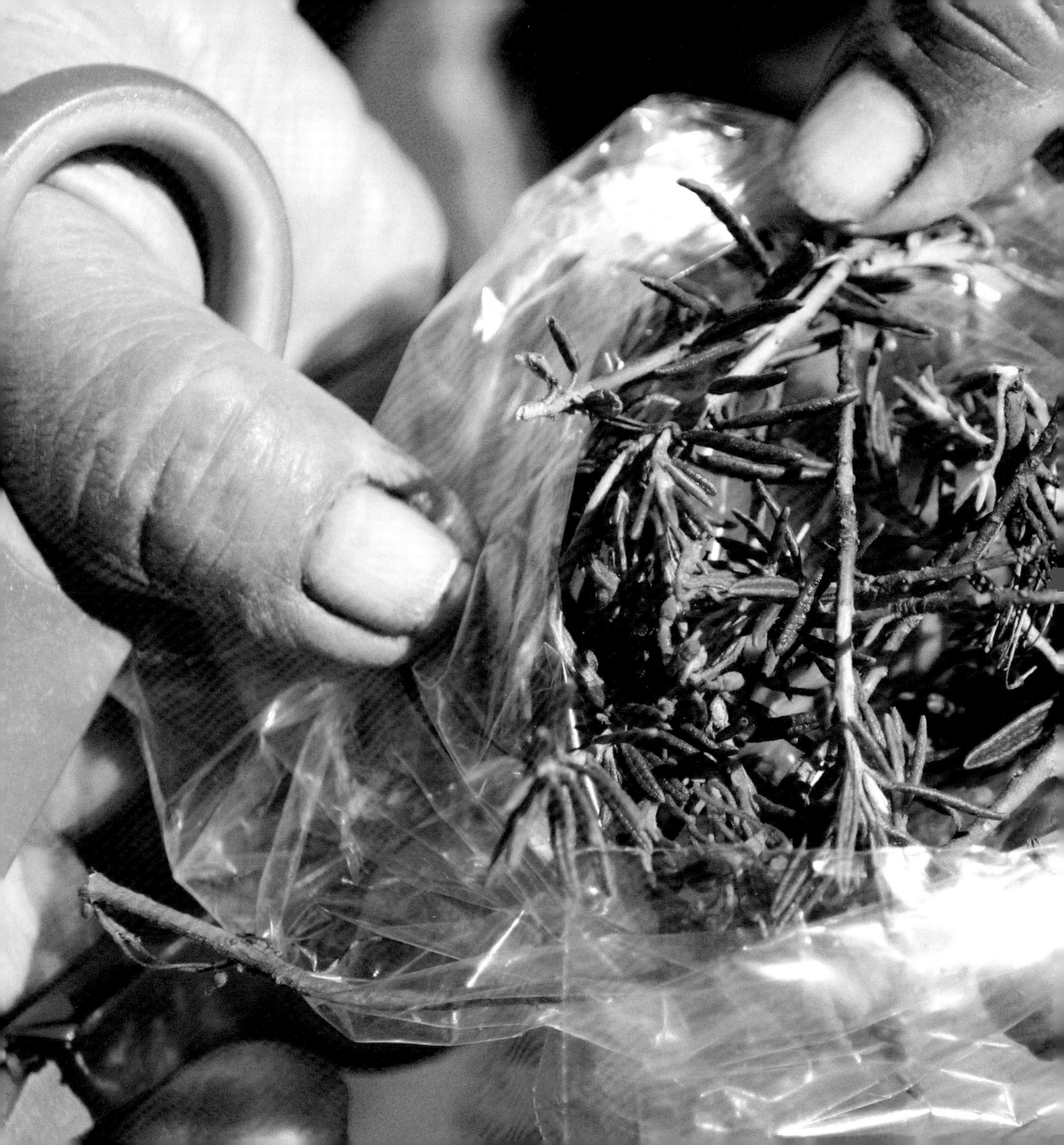

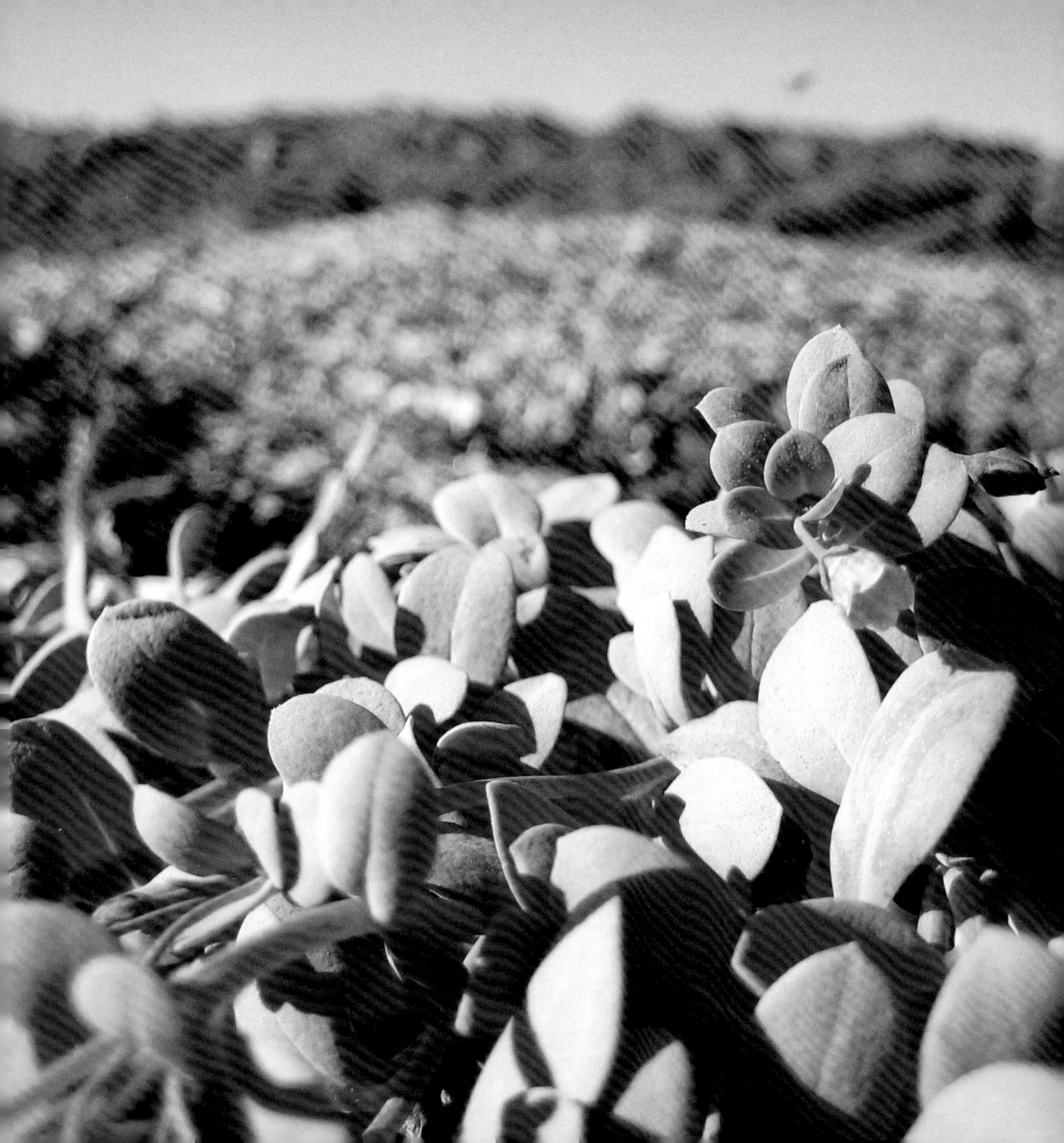

ᓯᐅᕋᐅᑉ ᐅᖃᐅᔭᖕᒋᑦ
Siuraup Uqaujangit / Seaside Bluebells

ᓯᐅᕋᐅᑉ ᐅᖃᐅᔭᖕᒋᑦ ᓯᔾᔭᒦᓰᑦ. ᐅᖃᐅᔭᖕᒋᑦ ᐊᓘᑎᑎᑐᑦ ᒥᒃᓯᖃᖅᑐᑎᑦ ᓯᐊᕐᓇᕈᔫᑦᑐᑎᒃ ᑐᖕᒍᔪᖅᑕᐅᓪᓗᑎᒃ ᐊᒻᒪᓗ ᕿᓪᓕᕋᑎ. ᓯᓕᓐᓂᖕᒋᑦ 3–5 ᒥᓕᒦᑐᒦᖃᑦᑕᖅᑐᑦ. ᐱᕈᖅᓯᐊᕌᔾᔪᑯᓗᖕᒋᑦ ᑐᖕᒍᔪᕈᔪᑦᑐᑯᓘᖃᑦᑕᖅᑐᑦ, ᓯᕙᓂᕈᑎᑎᑐᑦ ᒥᒃᓯᖃᖅᑐᑎᒃ. ᓯᐅᕋᐅᑉ ᐅᖃᐅᔭᖕᒋᑦ ᑕᑭᓪᓕᓗᐊᕈᓐᓇᖕᒋᑦᑐᑦ, ᑭᓯᐊᓂᑦ ᓇᑲᖕᒋᑦ 30 ᓯᐊᓐᑎᒦᑐᓂᑦ ᑕᑭᓂᖃᓕᓰᑦ.

Siuraup uqaujangit (seaside bluebells) grow in tufts on ocean beaches. The spoon-shaped leaves are light grey green and they are matte (not shiny). They are usually 3 mm to 5 mm thick. The little flowers are light blue, shaped like tiny bells. Siuraup uqaujangit does not grow tall, but its stems can grow up to 30 cm horizontally.

ᓯᐅᕋᐅᑉ ᐅᖃᐅᔭᖕᒋᑦ ᓴᖖᒋᓗᐊᕋᑎᑦ ᒪᒪᖅᑐᑯᓗᐃᑦ. ᓰᕐᓇᕈᔪᑦᑐᑎᒃ ᐊᕿᑦᑐᑯᓘᑦᓗᑎᒃ ᐊᒻᒪ ᐃᒃᓯᖃᑦᑎᐊᖅᑐᑎᒃ. ᐋᓚᓯᓕ ᐃᖅᑲᐅᒪᕗᖅ ᑕᐃᒪᐃᑦᑐᓂ ᓂᕇᓐᓇᕈᓐᓇᖃᑦᑕᓚᐅᕐᓂᖕᒐᓂᑦ ᓂᕕᐊᖅᓯᐊᖕᒍᑦᓗᓂ. ᐅᖃᐅᔭᖕᒋᑦ, ᐱᕈᖅᓯᐊᖕᒐ, ᐊᐃᕋᖕᒋᓐᓄᑦ ᓂᕆᔭᒃᓴᐃᓐᓇᐅᕗᑦ. ᒪᒪᕐᓂᖅᐹᖕᒍᕙᓪᓚᐃᔪᖅ ᐳᑯᑐᐃᓐᓇᕆᐊᖕᒐ, ᖃᓄᐃᓕᖕᒋᑦᑎᐊᕐᓗᒍ.

Siuraup uqaujangit is mild and pleasant to eat. It has a slight sweetness and is very tender and juicy. Aalasi recalls that there was no limit to how much she could eat of this plant as a child. The leaves, flowers, stems, and roots are all edible. The most delicious way to eat this plant is freshly picked, just as it is.

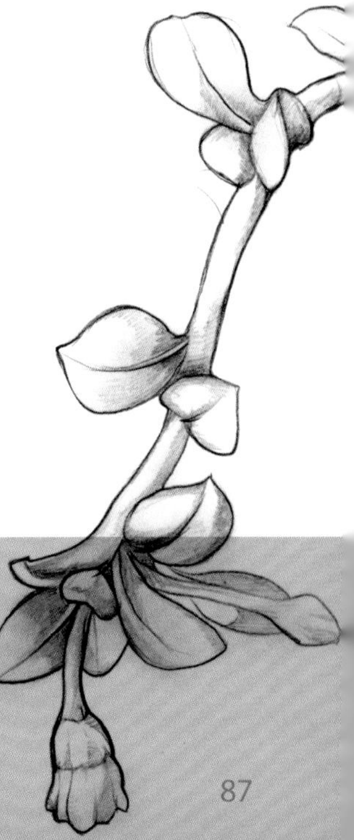

ᓯᐅᕋᐅᑉ ᐅᖃᐅᔭᖏᑦ ᒪᒪᖅᑐᐊᓘᒻᒥᔪᑦ ᐱᕈᖅᑐᕕᓂᕐᓂᑦ ᑐᖑᔪᖅᑕᓂᑦ ᐃᓚᓕᐅᑎᓗᒋᑦ, ᓵᕐᓗ ᐸᐅᓐᓇᓄᑦ (p. 47) ᐅᖔᓘᓐᓃᑦ ᖁᖑᓕᕐᓄᑦ (p. 55). ᐅᖃᐅᓯᖏᑦ ᓇᑲᖏᑦᓗ ᐃᓚᓕᐅᕝᓴᐅᔪᓐᓇᕐᒥᔪᑦ ᐃᖃᓗᕕᓂᐅᑉ ᖃᔪᖓᓄᑦ. ᐊᒃᑐᒐᓛᓚᐅᕐᓗᒋᑦ ᖃᔪᕐᒧᑦ ᐃᓚᓕᐅᑎᓗᒋᑦ ᐃᖃᓗᕕᓂᖅᑕᖃᕈᓐᓂᖅᑎᑦᓗᒍ. ᐊᐃᕋᖏᑦᑕᐅᑉ ᓂᕆᔭᐅᔪᓐᓇᕐᒥᔪᑦ ᐆᓯᒪᓗᒋᑦ, ᑐᖅᑕᑎᑐᑦ (p. 61). ᑎᖅᑎᑎᓚᐅᑳᓗᒋᑦ ᕿᓚᒥᕈᓗᒃ ᐊᕿᑦᓕᒐᔭᖅᑐᑦ ᓴᙱᓗᐊᕈᓐᓃᕐᓗᑎᑦᓗ.

Siuraup uqaujangit is also delicious mixed with other greens, such as *paunnait* (dwarf fireweed; p. 47) or *qunguliit* (mountain sorrel; p. 55). The leaves and stems can also be used to season and enrich fish broth. Chop them into small pieces and add them to the broth that remains after the boiled fish has been removed. The roots can also be eaten lightly cooked, as with *tuqtait* (alpine bistort rhizomes; p. 61). Cook them briefly in boiling water and they will become mild and tender.

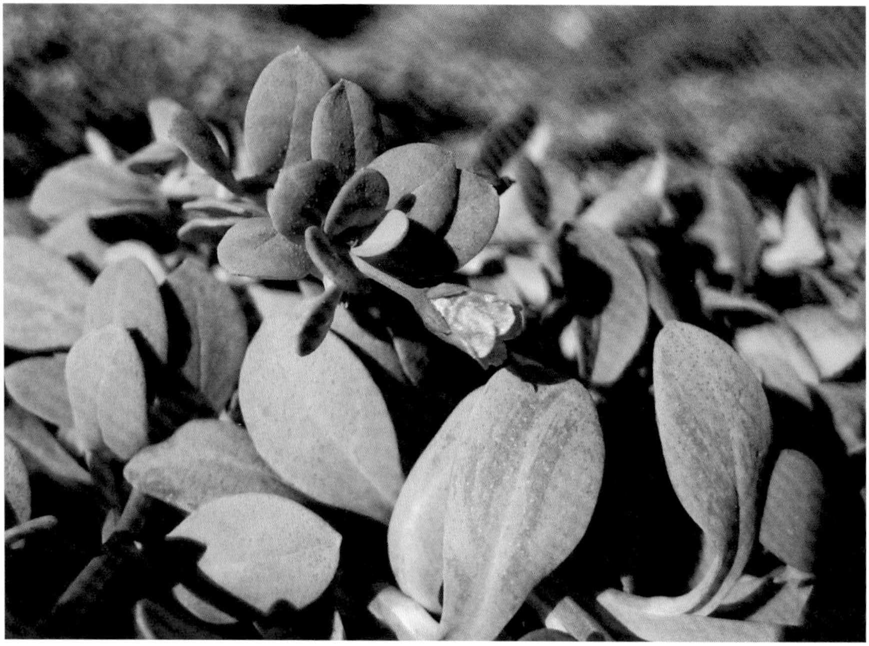

ᓯᐅᕋᐅᑉ ᐅᖃᐅᔮᖏᑦ ᐊᑲᐅᓯᓴᐅᑎᐅᔪᓐᓇᕐᒥᔪᑦ. ᐸᓐᓂᖅᑑᒥᑦ ᐊᕐᓇᕐᒥᑦ ᐊᐅᖏᕈᑎᔪᖅᑲᓚᐅᖅᓯᒪᒻᒪᑦ. ᐋᓚᓯᐅᑉ ᐊᓈᓇᖓᑕ ᓂᓇᑎᖖᒋᖕᒫᖅᑐᓂᐅᑉ ᓯᐅᕋᐅᑉ ᐅᖃᐅᔮᖓᓂ ᖃᔪᖅᑐᖅᑎᖃᑦᑕᓚᐅᖅᓯᒪᕚ. ᐊᑯᓂᐅᖏᑦᑐᖅ, ᐊᕐᓇᖅ ᐊᑲᐅᓯᔪᕕᓂᖅ. ᑏᖖᒍᐊᓕᐅᕐᓂᐊᕐᓗᓂ, ᐅᖃᐅᔮᖏᑦ ᓇᑲᖏᑦᓗ ᕿᓚᒥᑯᓗᒃ ᑎᖅᑎᑦᑐᒦᑎᒋᐊᓕᑦ, ᓴᖖᒋᔫᒻᒪᓇᐅᒻᒪᑕ.

Siuraup uqaujangit also has medicinal properties. There was once a woman in Pangnirtung who had lost a lot of blood. Aalasi's mother replaced the woman's meals with tea made from siuraup uqaujangit. After a short while, the woman recovered. To make tea from siuraup uqaujangit, boil the leaves and stems only briefly, as they are strong in flavour when boiled.

ᐱᕈᖅᓯᐊᕌᖅᔪᑯᓗᖏᑦ ᓯᐅᕋᐅᑉ ᐅᖃᐅᔮᖏᑦ ᕿᓚᒥᑯᓗᒃ ᓴᖅᑭᔩᑲᐃᓐᓇᓲᑦ ᐊᐅᔭᐅᑉ ᕿᑎᐊᒍ ᐱᑕᖅᑲᕈᓐᓃᓈᖅᑲᑦᑕᖅᑐᑦ.

The tiny blossoms of siuraup uqaujangit appear briefly in midsummer and then disappear.

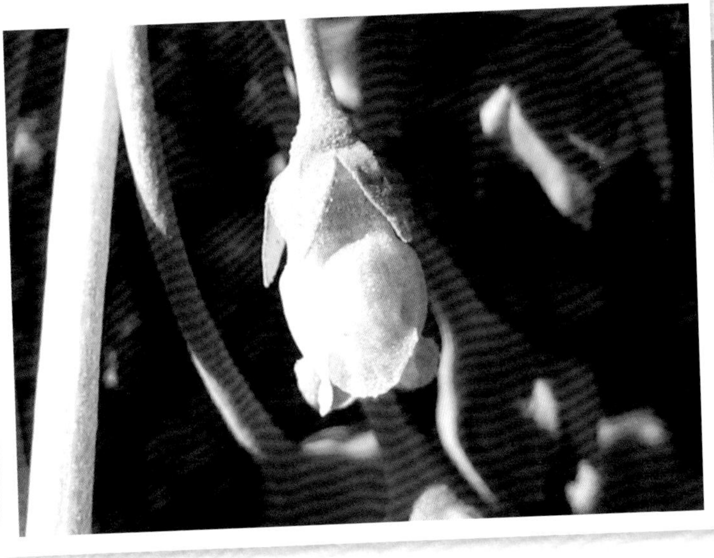

ᐃᑦᑎᓇᖅᑐᖅ ᐃᖃᓗᕕᓂᐅᑉ ᖃᔪᖓ ᓯᐅᕋᐅᑉ ᐅᖃᐅᔾᔨᖕᓂᑦ ᐃᓚᓕ
Savoury Char Broth with Siuraup Uqaujangit

- 1 ᐃᕐᖑᓯᖅ ᓯᐅᕋᐅᑉ ᐅᖃᐅᔾᔨᑦ, ᐊᒃᑐᒪᓵᔅᓯᒪᔪᑦ
- ᐃᖃᓗᕕᓂᐅᑉ ᖃᔪᖓ

- 1 cup of siuraup uqaujangit, chopped into small pieces
- Pot of cooking water from boiled fish

ᐃᖃᓗᓕᐅᕐᕕᕖᓃᑦ ᖃᔪᖓ (ᐃᑎᐅᔭᖅᑲᕈᓇᖅᑐᖅ ᐋᒃᑲᓘᓐᓃᑦ). ᖃᔪᖅ ᐆᓇᕐᓂᖓᓂ, ᓯᐅᕋᐅᑉ ᐅᖃᐅᔾᔨᑦ ᐊᒃᑐᒪᓵᒃᓯᒪᔪᑦ ᐃᓚᓕᐅᑎᓗᒋᑦ. ᐃᖑᓚᕐᓗᒍ ᐃᑲᕐᕋᖑᐊᒥᑦ ᐊᑕᐅᓯᕐᒥᑦ ᐊᒻᒪ ᖃᔪᖅᑐᖅᑎᐊᓕᕐᒥᓗᑎᑦ!

Save the cooking water from a pot of boiled char (with or without onions). While the water is still hot, add a generous handful of the chopped leaves and stems of siuraup uqaujangit. Stir the mixture for a minute or so and enjoy!

ᖃᐅᔨᒪᔭᕆᐊᓕᒃ: ᓯᐅᕋᐅᑉ ᐅᖃᐅᔾᔨᑦ ᓴᙱᔫᒪᕆᐅᒪᑕ ᖃᔪᖅᑐᕐᓇᓵᖅᑕᐃᓕᒍ ᕿᑲᑖᑦᑎᑦᑕᐃᓕᐅᑉ ᓴᙱᓗᐊᓕᑐᐃᓐᓇᕆᐊᖃᕐᒪᑦ.

Note: Siuraup uqaujangit is potent, so do not wait too long to drink the broth or the flavour may become too strong.

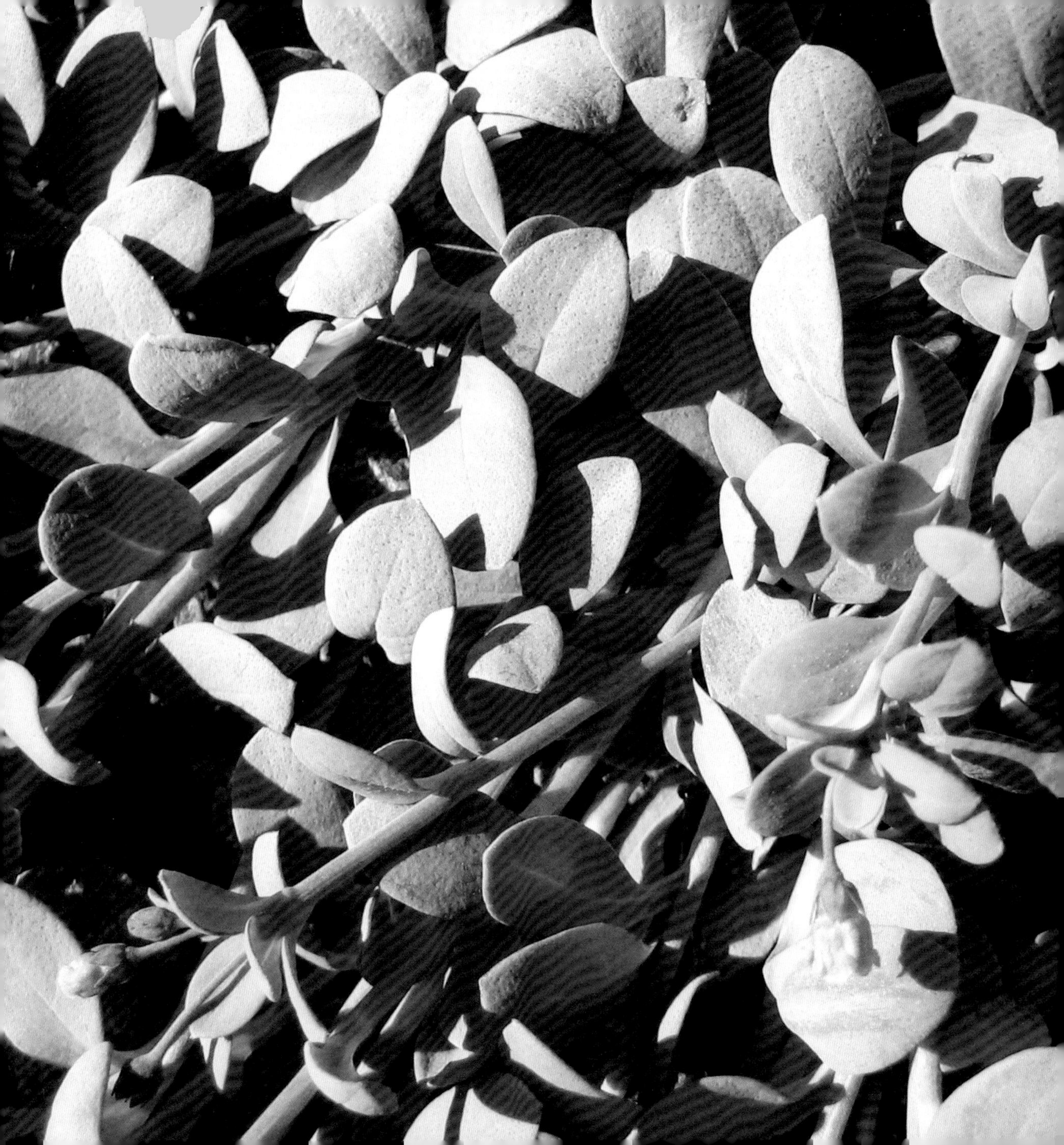

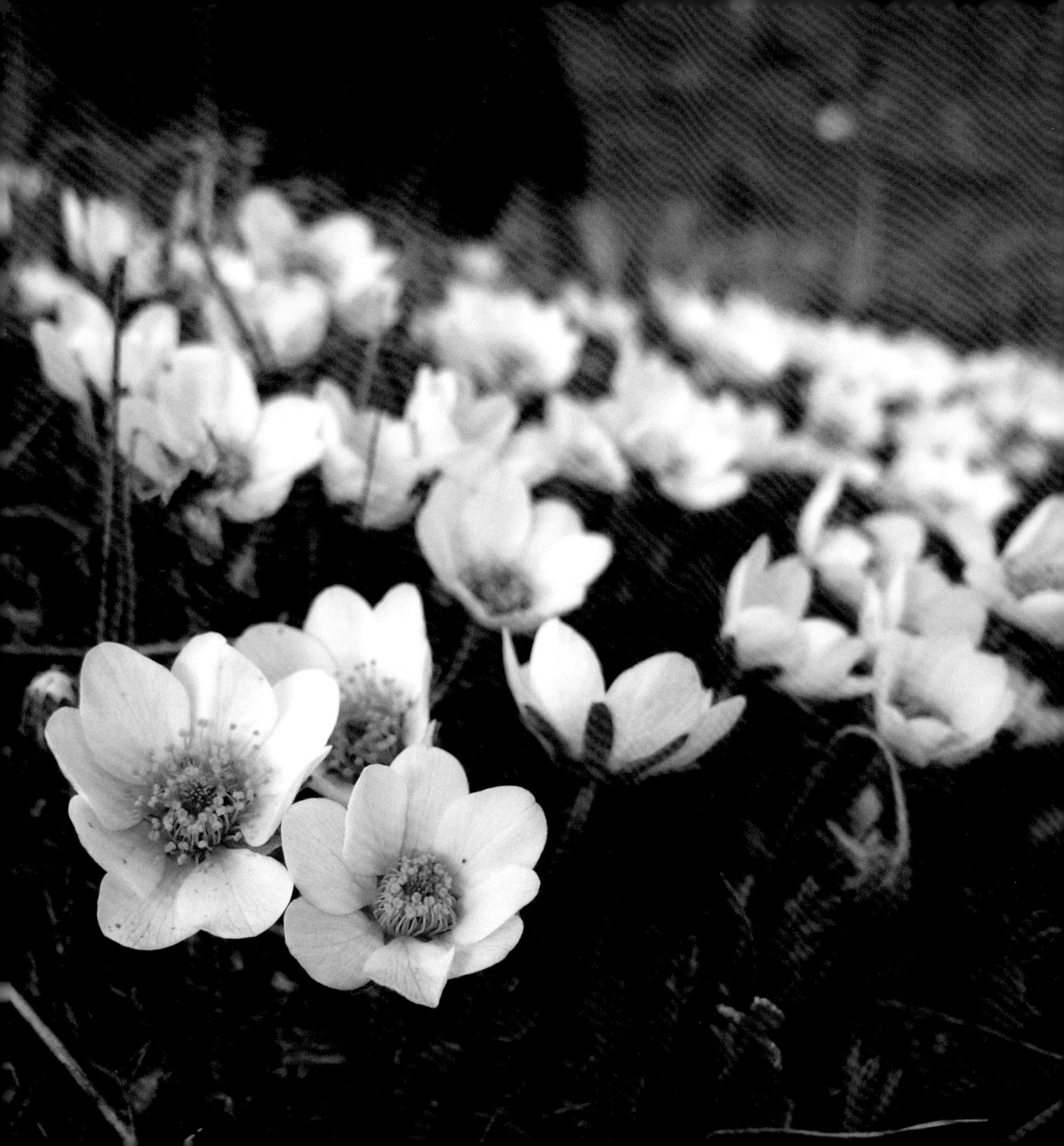

ᒪᓕᒃᑳᑦ
Malikkaat / Mountain Avens

ᒪᓕᒃᑳᑦ ᓄᓇᕋᖅᑖᓲᖑᕗᑦ ᔫᓐ ᐊᒻᒪᓗ ᔪᓚᐃ ᓄᖖᒍᐊᓂ. ᒪᓕᒃᑳᑦ ᖃᑯᖅᑕᐅᖃᑦᑕᖅᑐᑦ ᖁᖅᓱᖅᑐᓂᑦ ᕿᑎᖃᖅᑐᑎᑦ. ᐊᒻᒪᓗᖅᑐᑯᓘᔪᑦ ᑖᒃᑯᐊ. ᒪᓕᒃᑳᑦ ("ᒪᓕᑦᑏᑦ") ᓯᕿᓂᕐᒧᑦ ᓵᖖᒐᓲᑦ, ᐅᓪᓗᑕᒫᑦᑎᐊᖅ ᐃᖏᕐᕋᓂᖓᓂᑦ ᒪᓕᖃᑦᑕᖅᑐᑦ. ᓇᑲᖏᑦ ᒥᖅᑯᕈᔪᖃᖅᑐᑎᒃ ᐊᒻᒪ ᐅᖃᐅᔭᖃᕋᑎᒃ, ᑕᑭᓂᖃᖑᔪᑦ 4–12 ᓯᐊᓐᑎᒦᑕᓂᑦ. ᓄᓇᐅᑉ ᐊᑖᒎᖅᓯᒪᔪᓂᒃ ᐊᒫᕐᓂᑦ ᐱᕈᖃᑦᑕᖅᑐᑦ ᓴᒃᑯᖖᒍᐊᕋᓛᑯᓘᔮᖃᑦᑕᖅᑐᑦ.

Malikkaat (mountain avens, singular: malikkaaq) flower in late June or July. The flowers are creamy white with yellow centres. They are shaped like tiny satellite dishes. Malikkaat ("the one that follows") turn to face the sun, following it across the sky all day. The flowering stems are hairy and leafless. They are usually 4 cm to 12 cm high. The leaves grow on stems along the ground and are shaped like small arrowheads.

ᐱᕈᖅᓯᐊᖏᑦ ᐱᕈᓚᐅᖅᑎᓪᓗᒋᑦ, ᒥᖅᑯᖅᑖᖃᑦᑕᖅᑐᑦ ᓂᒪᐅᑎᓯᒪᔪᑯᓗᓐᓂᒃ ᕿᑎᐊᓂᖖᒎᖅᑐᓂᒃ ᓇᑉᐸᖓᔪᓂᒃ. ᐅᑭᐊᒃᓴᓕᖅᑎᓪᓗᒍ, ᐱᕈᖅᓯᐊᖏᑦ ᑲᑕᒐᖃᑦᑕᖅᑐᑦ ᐊᒻᒪᓗ ᒥᖅᑯᑯᓗᖏᑦ ᐸᓂᖄᖓᑕ ᓂᒪᐅᑎᓯᒪᔪᓐᓃᖅᑐᑎᒃ ᐅᕐᕈᖓᓕᖃᑦᑕᖅᑐᑦ, ᐊᓄᓇᕐᒧᓗ ᑎᑦᑕᐅᑎᑕᐅᕙᑦᑐᑎᒃ.

After the plant flowers, hairs from the centre of the flower grow up into twisted spikes. Toward autumn, the petals fall away, the seeds ripen, and the hairs uncoil, spreading the seeds in the wind.

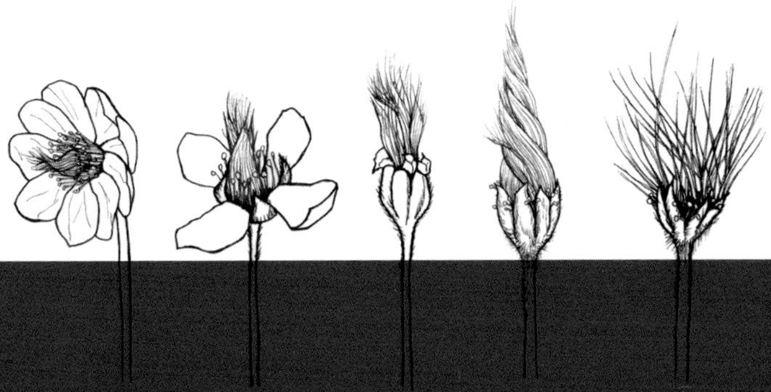

ᒪᓕᒃᑳᑦ ᖃᐅᔨᒪᔾᔪᑕᐅᔪᓐᓇᖅᑐᑦ ᓯᓚᒥᑦ. ᒥᖅᑯᖏᑦ ᓂᒪᐅᑎᓯᒪᔪᓐᓃᓕᖀᖕᒐᑕ, ᑕᐃᒪ ᐅᑭᐊᒃᓴᓕᕋᒥ ᐅᑭᐅᕐᒧᑐ ᐸᕐᓇᑉᐸᑦᑕᐊᓇᖅᓯᑦᑐᓂ. ᒪᓕᒃᑳᑦ ᓯᓚᐅᑉ ᖃᓄᐃᓐᓂᓇᓂᐊᖅᑕᖓᓂ ᖃᐅᔨᒪᔾᔪᑕᐅᔪᓐᓇᓇᕿᑦ. ᐱᕈᖅᓯᐊᑯᓗᖏᑦ ᓱᑲᖕᒐᖅᑰᔨᑦᑐᑎᒃ ᐃᓵᖕᒐᑦᑐᑎᒃ ᑲᑎᒻᒪᑦᑎᐊᖀᖕᒐᑕ, ᑕᐃᒪ ᑭᓯᐊᓂ ᓂᑦᓚᓱᓐᓂᐊᕿᒥ. ᐱᕈᖅᓯᐊᖏᑦᑐ ᖃᓱᖕᒐᑦᑐᑎᒃ ᒪᑉᐱᖕᒐᕐᑎᐊᖅᑎᑦᑐᑎᑦ, ᑕᐃᒪᒎᖅ ᓯᓚ ᐅᖅᑰᓂᐊᕿᒪᑦ.

Malikkaat can be used to judge the season. When the hairs start to uncoil, it is almost autumn and time to prepare for winter. Malikkaat can also be used to judge the weather. If the blossoms are tightly cupped, then the weather will be cold. If the blossoms are open and loose, the weather will be hot.

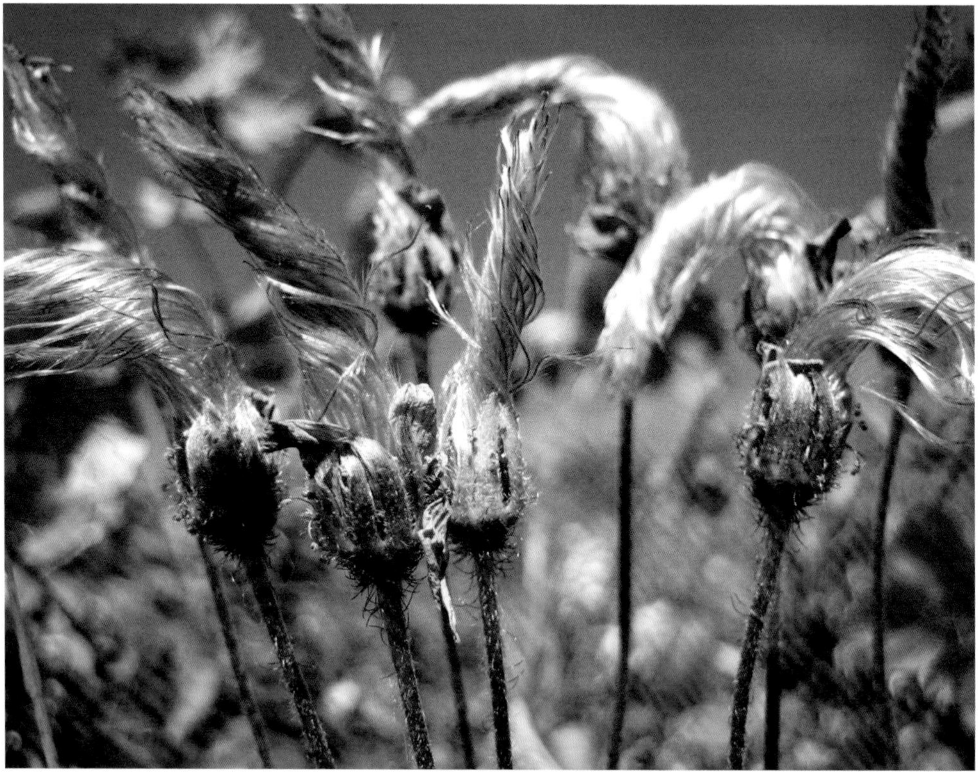

ᐊᔾᔨᓕᐅᕆᔪᕕᓂᖅ ᐃᐊᓚᓐ ᓯᒡᓗᕐ Photo by Ellen Ziegler

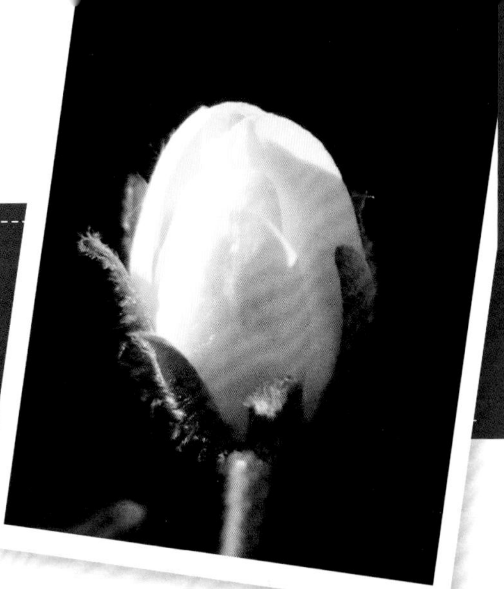

ᒪᓕᒃᑳᑦ ᐱᕈᓕᓱᑦ ᔪᓚᐃᕈᕋᑖᖅᑎᓪᓗᒍ.

Malikkaaq bud in early July.

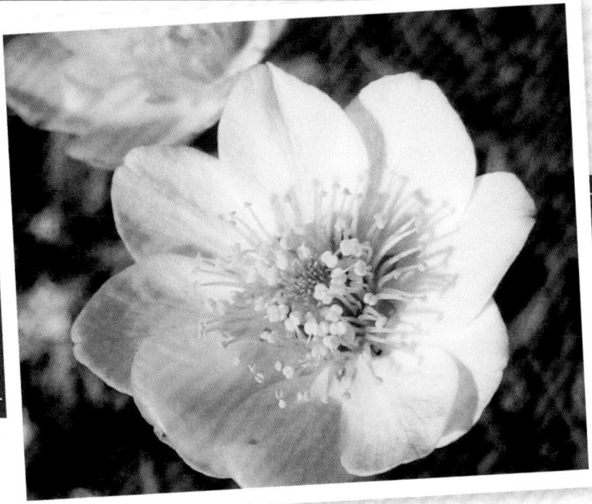

ᒪᓕᒃᑳᑦ ᔪᓚᐃ ᕿᑎᐊᓂᑦ ᐱᕈᓃᖅᑐᖅ.

Malikkaaq blossom in mid-July.

ᒪᓕᒃᑳᑦ ᐋᒡᒌᓯᐅᑉ ᕿᑎᐊᓂᑦ. ᒥᖅᑯᖏᑦ ᕿᑎᐊᓃᑦᑐᑦ
ᐃᒧᕙᑦᓯᐊᓕᖅᑎᕐᓗᑎᑦ.

Malikkaaq blossom in mid-August. The hairs are beginning to coil up at the centre.

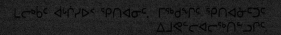

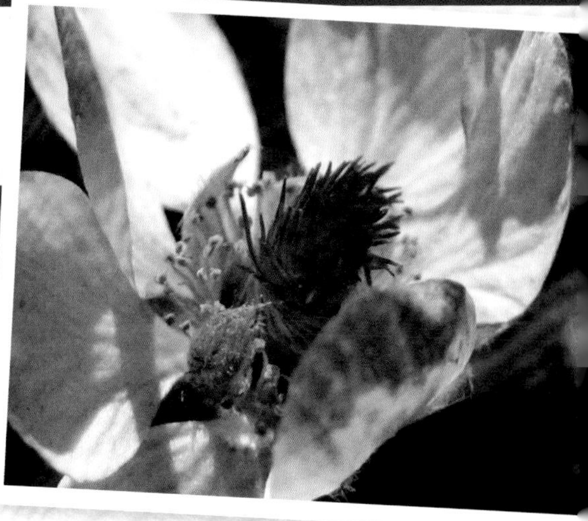

ᒪᓕᒃᑳᑦᑕᐅᖅ ᖃᐅᔨᒪᔾᔭᑕᐅᔪᓐᓇᕆᕗᑦ ᓇᓕᐊᓐᓄᑦ ᑐᕌᕆᐊᖅᑲᕐᒪᖔ ᐊᖏᕐᕋᕋᓱᒃᑐᑦ ᐃᓄᒃ ᑕᒃᓯᓕᐅᔾᔭᐅᓯᒪᔪᖅ ᐅᕝᕙᓘᓐᓃᑦ ᑖᖅᓯᔪᐊᓘᓐᓂᕈᓂ. ᐱᕈᖅᓯᐊᖑᓂᖓ ᓯᕿᓂᕐᒧᑦ ᓵᙵᑐᐅᔭᐃᓐᓇᕐᒪᑦ, ᓇᒦᓲᖑᒻᒪᖔ ᖃᐅᔨᒪᒍᕕᐅ ᓯᕿᓂᖅ ᖃᖓᒃᑯᑦ, ᖃᐅᔾᔭᐅᑎᒋᔪᓐᓇᕋᔭᖅᑕᑎᑦ, ᓇᓕᐊᓐᓄᑦ ᓵᙵᓗᑎᑦ ᐱᓯᒋᐊᖅᑲᕐᒪᖔᖅᐱᑦ.

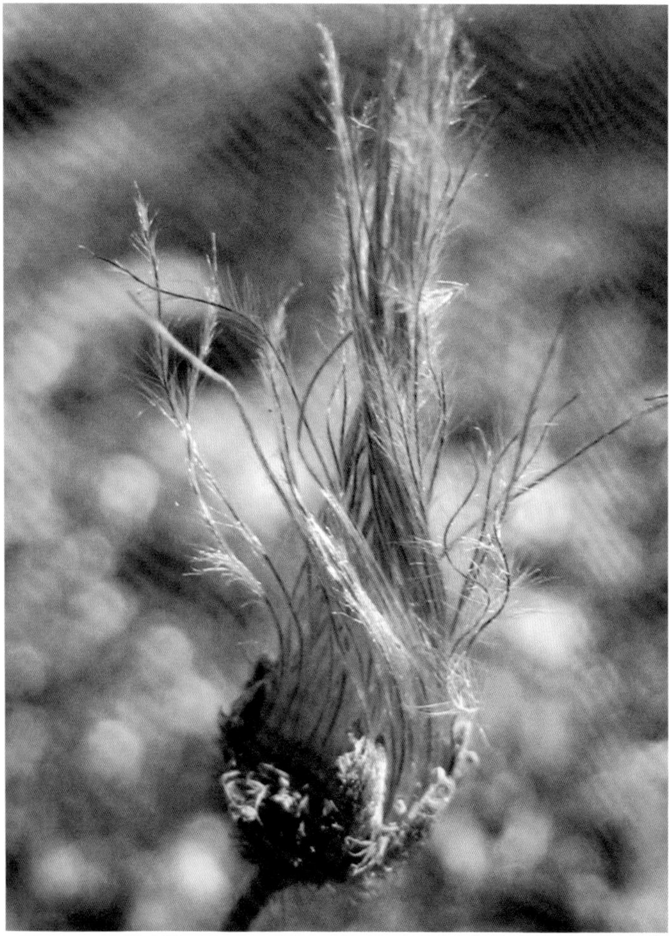

Malikkaat can also help someone if they are lost in fog or if it is dark and they cannot see their way home. The buds and flowers always turn to face the sun, so if you are familiar with the sun's location in relation to your home, you will know which direction to take.

ᐃᑲᔪᕐᓂᖅᑲᕐᓂᖏᓐᓄᑦ ᒪᓕᒃᑳᑦ, ᐃᓄᐃᑦ ᐅᖅᑲᐅᔾᔭᐅᖅᑲᑦᑕᖅᑐᕕᓃᑦ ᐲᔭᓇᓗᑎᒃ ᑐᑦᑕᕋᖅᑲᑦᑕᕐᑯᔭᐅᓇᑎᒃ. ᐊᒻᒪᑦᑕᐅ, ᐊᕐᓇᐃᑦ ᐃᕐᓂᑕᕌᖓᑕ, ᐋᑕᓯ ᐃᖅᑲᐅᒪᒻᒥᔪᖅ ᖃᐅᔨᖅᑲᑦᑕᓚᐅᖅᓯᒪᒐᒥ

ᒪᓕᒃᑳᑦ ᐃᒧᔨᒪᔪᓐᓃᖅᐸᑦᑕᐊᔪᖅ ᓲᑎᐱᓇᐅᑉ ᐱᒋᐊᕐᓂᖓᓂᑦ.

Malikkaaq beginning to uncoil in early September.

ᐃᕐᓂᐊᖑᔫᑉ ᓂᐊᕐᖁᖓ ᒪᓕᒃᑳᓄᑦ ᐅᐃᔾᔭᓪᓚᒃᑎᑕᐅᕐᑲᑦᑕᕐᓂᕐᒪᑕ ᐃᕐᓂᓯᒃᓲᔪᓄᑦ, ᓱᕐᑭᓂᐅᑉ ᐃᖏᕐᕋᓂᖓᓄ (ᓱᕐᑭᙳᔭᐅᑉ ᐅᐃᔾᔮᕐᓂᖓ ᒪᓕᒃᑐᒍ).

Because malikkaat are so helpful, people are told not to step on them or destroy them on purpose. Aalasi recalls that when women had babies, it was common for midwives to take the baby's head and gently turn it in the direction of malikkaat, toward the sun (clockwise).

ᓇᑲᖓᑕ ᒥᖅᑯᕈᔪᖏᑦ ᐊᑐᕐᓗᒋᑦ ᐃᔨᑎᕈᑎᒥᔭᐅᕐᑲᑦᑕᕐᓂᓀᕗᑦ. ᑕᐃᒫᑦᓕ ᐊᑐᖅᑕᐅᓂᐊᖅᑎᓪᓗᒋᑦ, ᒪᓕᒃᑳᑦ ᐃᖏᕐᕋᓂᓀᕐᑲᑦᑕᖅᑕᖓ ᒪᓕᒃᑐᒍ ᐅᐃᔾᔭᓪᓚᒃᑎᑕᐅᕐᑲᑦᑕᕐᓂᓀᕗᑦ.

The hairs on the stems of malikkaat may be used like tiny cloths to clean an irritation from an eye. When using the stems this way, they are to be turned in the direction that the malikkaat turn to follow the sun.

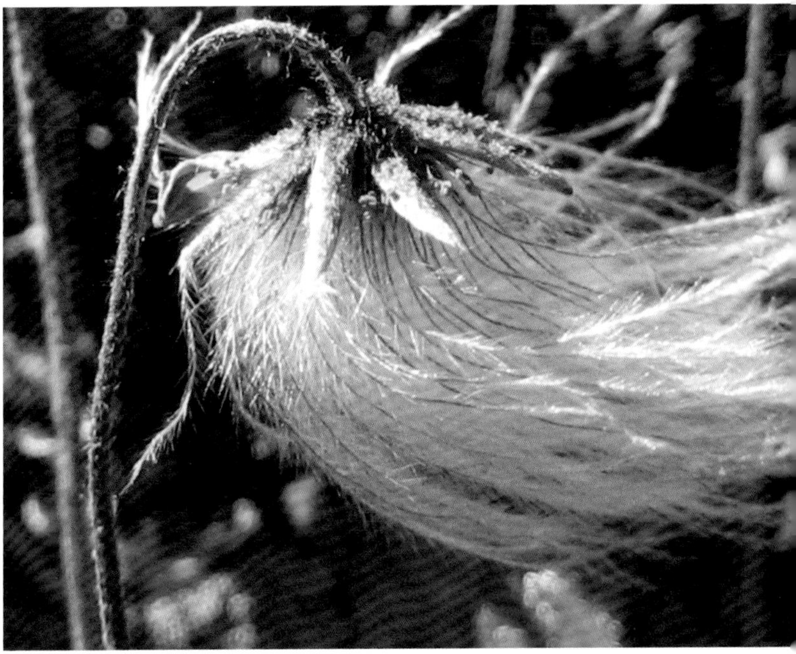

ᒪᓕᒃᑳᑦ ᐃᒍᓯᒪᖏᑦᑎᐊᓕᖅᑐᖅ ᐅᑭᐊᒃᓴᖅᑎᓪᓗᒍ, ᐊᐱᓂᐊᑦᑎᐊᓕᖅᑎᓪᓗᒍ.

Malikkaaq fully uncoiled in autumn, just before the first snowfall.

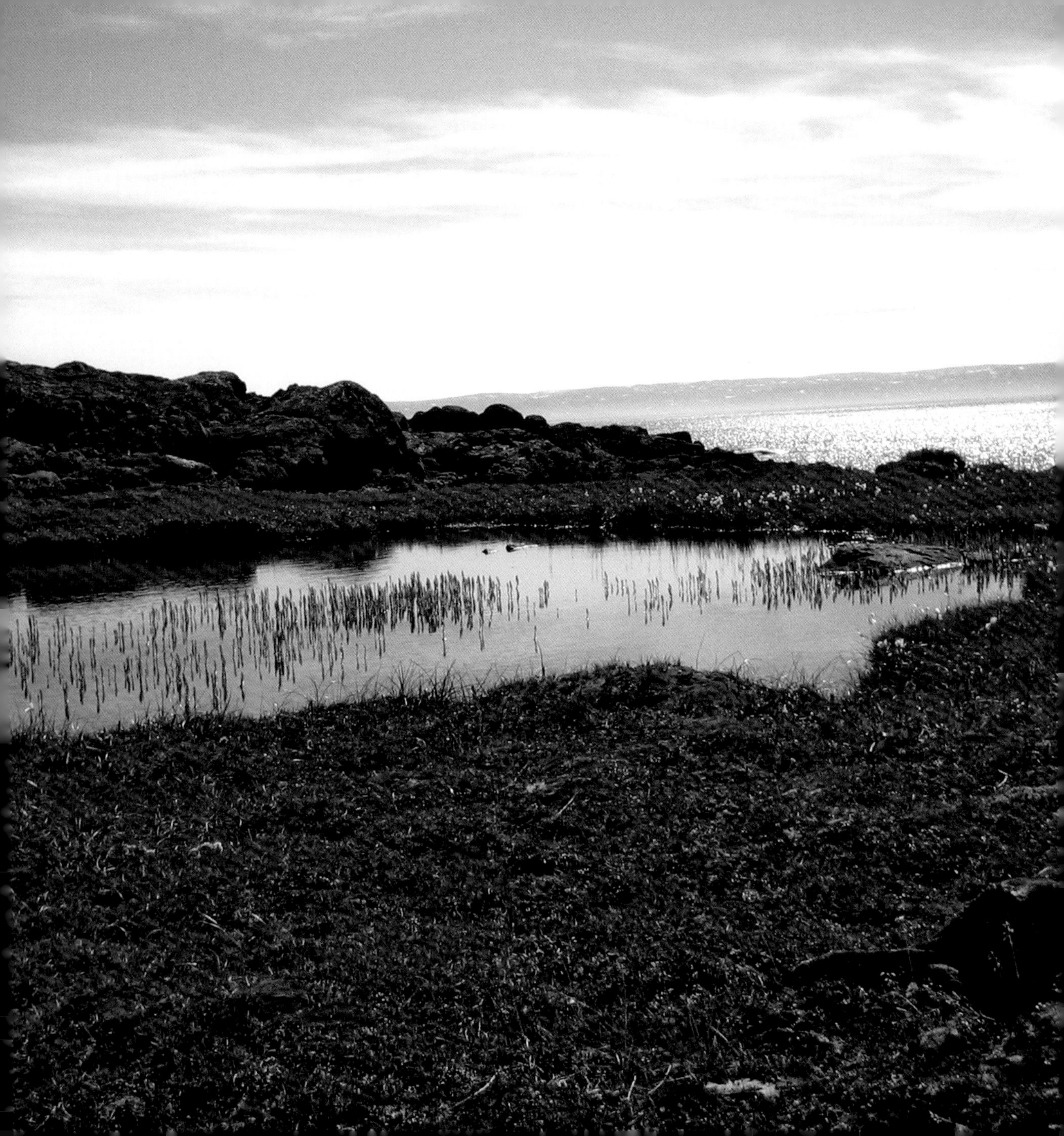

ᐅᕐᔪ

Urju / Peat Moss

ᐅᕐᔪ ᐱᑕᕐᑲᒐᔪᒃᑐᑦ ᑕᓯᐅᔭᐃᑦ ᑭᑦᑕᙱᓐᓂᑦ ᐊᒻᒪᓗ ᒪᓴᕐᓗᒻᒥᑦ, ᐱᓗᐊᖅᑐᒥᑦ ᓄᓇᕗᑦ ᐅᖅᑯᖅᐸᓯᖕᒐᓂᑦ. ᐱᕈᖅᑲᑦᑕᖅᑐᑦ ᒪᓴᕈᔪᒻᒥᑦ, ᓄᓇᓂᑦ ᐊᕐᑭᑦᑐᓂᑦ. ᐊᒥᐊᖅᑲᓲᖑᓪᓗᑎᑦ ᑲᔪᕐᓂᑦ, ᑐᖑᔪᖅᑕᓂᑦ, ᖁᖅᓱᖅᑐᓂᑦ ᐊᒻᒪᓗ ᖃᑯᕈᔪᒃᑐᓂᑦ.

Urju (peat moss) is common around the edges of ponds and in other wet areas of the tundra, especially in the southern parts of Nunavut. It grows in moist, spongy mats. Its colour ranges from brown and green to yellow and creamy white.

ᐅᕐᔪ ᓴᓗᒻᒪᖅᓴᐅᑎᖅᑲᖅᐳᑦ ᐊᒻᒪ, ᐸᓂᖅᑎᓯᒪᓪᓗᒋᑦ ᐃᒃᓯᑳᒃᑲᓐᓂᕈᓐᓇᖅᑐᑎᑦ ᐊᓪᓚᕈᑎᒋᓗᒋᑦ. ᑕᐃᒫ, ᐊᑑᑎᓪᓚᒻᒪᕆᐅᕗᑦ.

Urju has natural antiseptic properties and when it is dried, it is highly absorbent. So, it has many practical uses.

ᐋᓚᓯ ᐃᖅᑲᐅᒪᕗᑦ ᐃᓚᒌᑦ ᐊᖏᔪᒻᒪᕆᓐᓂᑦ ᓄᐊᑦᑎᖅᑲᑦᑕᓚᐅᖅᓯᒪᒐᒥᑦ ᐅᑭᐅᒃᑯᑦ ᐃᓕᒃᑯᐊᔅᓴᖕᒋᓐᓂᒃ. ᐅᕐᔪ ᐸᓂᖅᓯᐊᕆᔭᐅᖅᑲᑦᑕᓚᐅᖅᓯᒪᔪᑦ ᐊᑐᕆᐊᖅᑲᓚᕌᖓᑕ ᐊᑐᐃᓐᓇᐅᓂᐊᖅᒪᑕ. ᐸᓂᖅᓲᓂᐊᖅᑐᓂ ᐅᕐᔪᓂᑦ, ᓄᐊᑦᑎᓚᐅᖅᑐᑎᑦ ᐅᔭᕋᐃᑦ ᖄᖓᓄᑦ ᐅᕝᕙᓘᓐᓃᑦ ᐸᓂᖅᑐᒧᑦ ᐃᓕᐅᖅᑐᕈᓐᓇᖅᑕᑎᑦ. ᑕᐃᒪᙵᓕᒫᐸᓗᒃ, ᐅᑦᓗᐃᓐᓇᖅ ᐸᓂᕋᓱᓲᑦ. ᐅᕐᔪ ᐸᓂᖅᑎᓯᒪᓪᓗᒋᑦ ᓂᕈᒥᑦᑎᕆᔪᑦ ᐅᑲᓕᐅᑉ ᒥᖅᑯᖓᑎᑦ.

Aalasi recalls her family collecting large quantities of urju in the summer to be used during the winter. The urju was dried and then stored in a place to which her family could return when they needed some. To dry urju, pick it from the ground and spread it across rocks or another dry surface. Normally, it will dry within a day. Dried urju is as soft as rabbit fur.

ᐸᓂᖅᑎᓯᒪᔪᑦ ᐅᕐᔪ ᖁᑦᑕᕐᕕᐅᔪᓐᓇᕐᒥᔪᑦ ᐅᕝᕙᓗᓐᓃᑦ ᐊᐅᓈᖅᑐᒧᑦ ᐊᑐᖅᑕᐅᔪᓐᓇᖅᑐᑎᒃ. ᖁᑦᑕᕐᕕᐅᓂᐊᖅᑎᓪᓗᒋᑦ ᐊᐅᓈᖅᑐᒧᓪᓘᓐᓂᑦ ᐊᑐᖅᑕᐅᓂᐊᖅᑎᓪᓗᒋᑦ, ᐋᓚᓯ ᐃᖅᑲᐅᒪᔪᖅ ᐸᓚᐅᒑᖅ ᐴᕕᓂᖕᒐᓂᑦ ᖄᖅᑲᖅᑎᑕᐅᖅᑲᑦᑕᓚᐅᕐᓂᖕᒋᓐᓂᒃ. ᐸᓚᐅᒑᖅ ᐴᕕᓂᖕᒋᑦ ᓂᕈᒥᒻᒪᑕ ᐅᐊᓴᕿᕐᓂᖅᑐᑎᓪᓗ. ᖁᑦᑕᕐᕕᓕᐅᕿᓯᒃᑐᓂᓕ ᖃᓪᓗᓈᖅᑕᖅ ᓴᓇᖅᑳᓚᐅᖅᑐᒍ ᐃᓗᑦᓕᕈᐃᓐᓇᖅᑲᑦᑕᖅᑕᕕᓂᖕᒋᑦ ᐅᕐᔪᓂᒃ. ᑎᒍᓯᓗᑎᑦ ᒪᕐᕿᐊᖅᑎᕐᓗᒍ ᐊᒡᒐᐃᑦ ᑕᑕᓪᓗᒍ ᐊᑕᐅᓯᕐᒧᑦ ᖁᑦᑕᕐᕕᒻᒧᑦ ᓈᒻᒪᖅᑲᑦᑕᖅᑐᕕᓂᖅ. ᐋᓚᓯ ᐃᖅᑲᐅᒪᔪᖅ ᐅᕐᔪ ᐊᑐᐃᓐᓇᐅᑎᓐᓇᒋᑦ ᐅᑲᓚᐅᑉ ᐊᒥᖕᒐᓂᑦ ᐊᑐᖅᑲᑦᑕᖅᑐᕕᓂᖅ, ᑭᓯᐊᓂ ᐅᕐᔪ ᐱᐅᒋᓂᖅᓴᓇᖅᑲᑦᑕᖅᑕᕕᓂᖕᒋᑦ

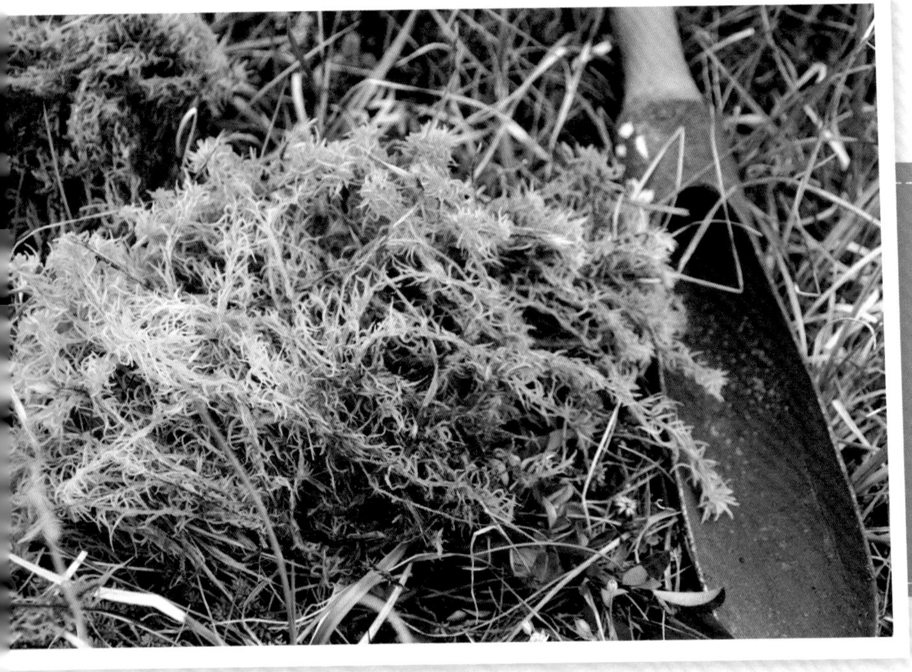

ᐋᓚᓯ ᖃᓄᕋᐅᑎᕋᓛᒧᑦ ᐲᖅᓯᔪᖅ ᐅᕐᔪᒥᑦ ᑕᓯᐅᑉ ᑭᓪᓚᖕᒐᓂᑦ.

Aalasi uses a small shovel to remove urju from the wet edges of a pond.

ᐃᒋᑐᐃᓐᓇᕿᒃᓴᐅᓂᖏᓐᓄᑦ ᐊᑐᓅᖅᑐᑎᑦ. ᐊᑦᓚᓯ ᐃᖅᑲᐅᒪᔪᖅ ᐅᕐᔪᐃᑦ ᐊᑦᑕᓂᑕᐊᖑᕐᑲᑦᑕᓚᐅᕐᓂᖏᓐᓂᑦ ᕐᑭᒻᒥᑖᓄᑦ, ᐊᑐᐃᓐᓇᕐᑲᐃᓐᓇᕈᔪᑉᐸᓚᐅᕐᒪᑕ ᐃᓚᒌᑦ. ᓱᕈᖀᖕᒐᑕᓕ ᐃᒋᑐᐃᓐᓇᕿᒃᓴᐅᕐᑲᑦᑕᕐᓂᕐᒪᑕ.

Dried urju can be used as a diaper or as a menstrual pad. To make a diaper or pad, Aalasi recalls using cotton flour bags because flour bags were soft and easy to wash. She would tie the flour bag on as a diaper and then stuff the bottom with urju. About two handfuls of urju is sufficient for one diaper. Aalasi recalls that if urju were unavailable, she used rabbit fur instead, but urju was preferable because it was discarded after one use.

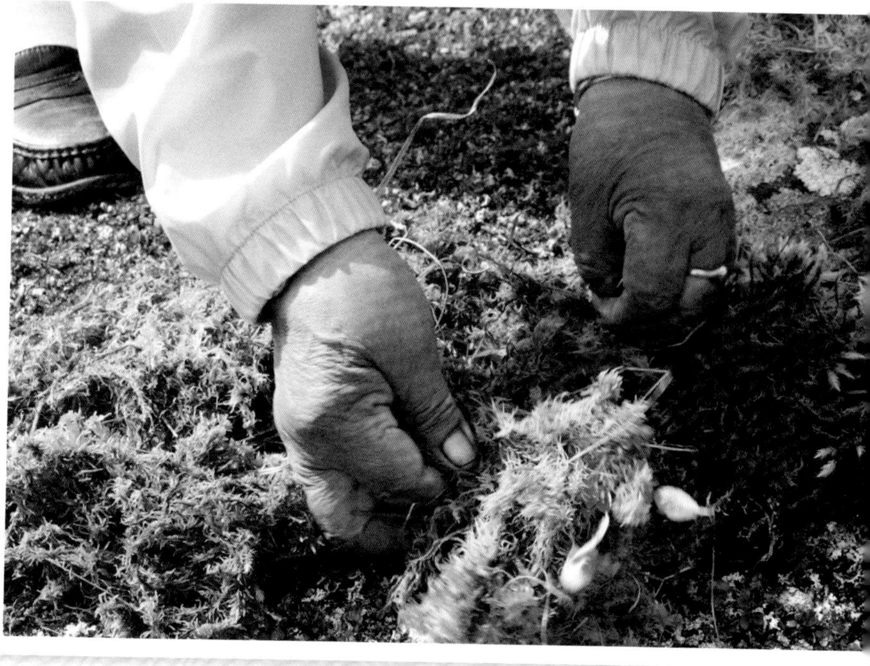

ᐋᓚᓯ ᐃᓯᕕᑎᓇᔪᖅ ᐅᕐᔪᖕᓂᒃ ᐃᓂᓚᐅᖕᒋᓐᓂᕐᓂᑦ ᐅᔭᕋᐅᑉ ᖄᖕᒐᓄᑦ ᐸᓂᖅᓯᐊᓇᓗᓂᒋᑦ.

Aalasi separates the urju before laying it out on a rock to dry.

Aalasi also remembers using dried urju as bedding for newborn puppies, which her family almost always had. The urju was simply tossed away when it was soiled.

ᐸᓂᖅᑎᓯᒪᔪᑦ ᐅᕐᔪᑦ ᐅᒃᓯᒃᓴᐅᑎᒋᔭᐅᔪᓐᓇᕆᕗᑦ ᑐᐱᕐᓄᑦ ᖃᕐᒪᕐᓄᓪᓗ. ᐊᓇᙵᕆᖅᑲᔾᔭᐃᒃᑯᑎᐅᔪᓐᓇᖅᑐᑎᒡᓗ ᑕᐃᒫ. ᐋᓚᓯ ᐃᖅᑲᐅᒪᔨᕗᖅ ᐊᖑᓇᓱᒃᑎᑦ ᑲᒥᒻᒥᓂᒃ ᐃᓗᓪᓕᖅᓯᐃᖅᑲᑦᑕᕐᓂᕐᒪᑕ ᐅᖅᑰᔾᔪᑎᒃᓴᒃᑲᓂᕐᓂᑦ.

Dried urju can be used around the edges of tents and qarmaqs for insulation. This may also help to keep insects out. Aalasi also recalls hunters adding extra insulation to their kamiit by stuffing dried urju into them.

ᐳᐊᓗᙳᐊᑦ (p. 23) ᐊᒻᒪ ᓱᐳᑎᑦ (ᒥᖅᑯᖓ ᓱᐳᑎᐅᑉ; p. 33) ᐱᑕᖃᙱᑉᐸᑕ ᐅᕐᔪ ᒪᓂᕆᔭᒃᓴᐅᒻᒥᔪᑦ. ᑭᓯᐊᓂ ᐃᒻᒥᒃᑯᑦ ᐃᑭᑦᑐᑎᑦ ᓄᙳᓴᕋᐃᑦᑐᑯᓘᒐᓗᐊᑦ, ᐊᑐᕋᒃᓴᐅᒐᓗᐊᖅᑐᑎᑦ. ᐱᐅᓂᖅᐹᖑᕗᖅᑕ ᐊᕝᕙᓗᐊᖓᓂ ᐃᓚᓗᒍ ᒪᓂᕐᒥᑦ (p. 29).

If *pualunnguat* (Arctic cotton; p. 23) and *suputit* (*uqpi suputillu*, Arctic willow; p. 33) are not available, urju can be used as a wick for a qulliq. It is not ideal as a wick because it burns too quickly, but it will suffice. It will burn best if combined, half and half, with *maniq* (lamp moss; p. 29).

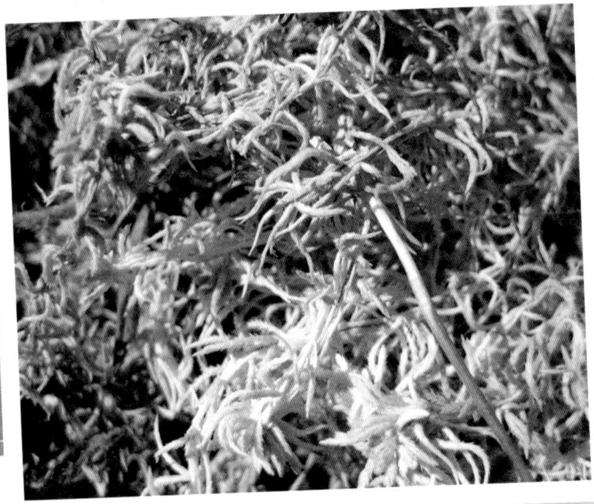

ᐅᕐᔪ ᐸᓂᖅᑐᕕᓂᖅ ᐅᓐᓄᐊᖕᒋᓐᓇᖅ. ᐅᕐᔪ ᓂᕈᒥᒃᑐᑯᓗᐃᑦ ᐸᓂᖅᑎᓯᒪᓪᓗᒋᑦ ᓲᕐᓗ ᐅᑲᓕᐅᑉ ᒥᖅᑯᖏᑎᑐᑦ.

Urju dried on a rock overnight. When urju is dried, it is as soft as rabbit fur.

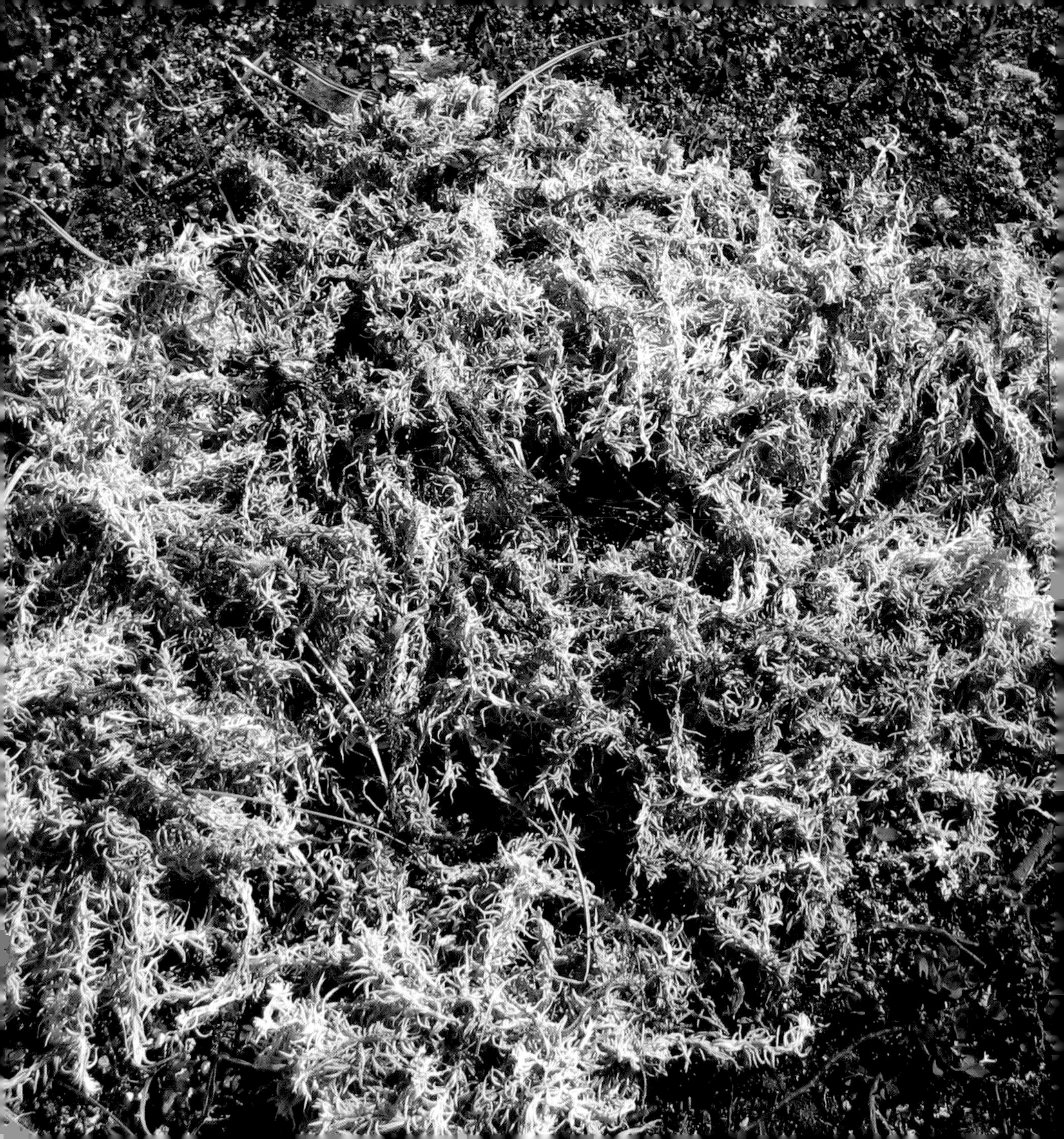

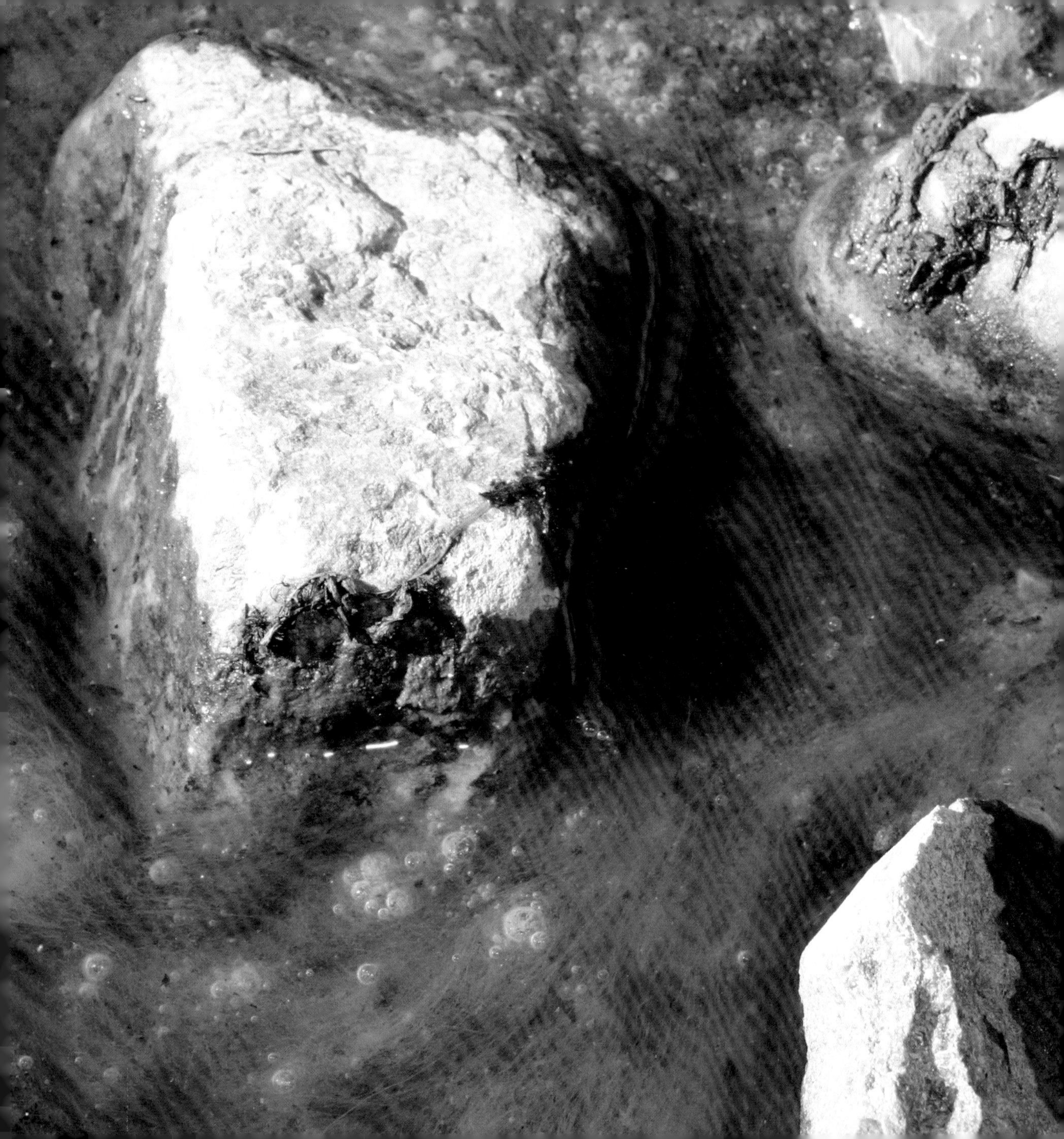

ᐃᔾᓯᐅᑎ
Ijisiuti / River Algae

ᐃᔾᓯᐅᑎ ᐱᕈᖅᑲᑦᑕᖅᑐᑦ ᑰᒐᓛᓂᒃ ᑰᖕᓂᑦᑐ ᓄᓇᕗᒻᒥᑦ. ᐊᒥᐊᖅᑲᖅᐸᑦᑐᑎᑦ ᑐᖑᔪᖅᑕᓂᑦ ᑕᖅᓴᐅᓕᓃᑦᑐᑎᑦ.

Ijisiuti (river algae) grows on rocks in many creeks and rivers across Nunavut. Its colour ranges from light to dark green and it is made up of many small strands.

ᐃᔾᓯᐅᑎ ᐊᑐᖅᑕᐅᔪᓐᓇᖅᑐᑦ ᐊᑲᐅᓯᓴᐅᑕᐅᔪᑎᒃ ᐃᔾᓄᑦ, ᐃᔾᐅᑉ ᓯᓚᑖᓄᑦ, ᐊᒻᒪ ᖁᕝᕕᐅᖅᕕᓄᑦ. ᐋᓚᓯᐅᑉ ᐊᖓᔪᖓ ᐃᔾᓄᒃᑐᕝᕕᓂᖅ ᒪᒃᑯᑦᑐᓂ. ᐃᔾᖓᓄᑦ ᐃᓕᓯᔪᖅᑲᓚᐅᖅᓯᒪᔪᖅ ᐃᔾᓯᐅᑎᒥᑦ ᐅᓐᓄᐊᓕᒫᖅ ᐊᑕᑎᑕᐅᓪᓗᓂ ᐃᔾᖓᓗ ᖃᓪᓗᓈᖅᑕᒥᑦ ᒪᑐᒻᒥᓪᓗᒍ. ᐃᔾᖓ ᐱᐅᓯᔫᖅᑐᕝᕕᓂᖅ.

Ijisiuti can be used as a medicinal eye ointment to help with eye, eyelid, and tear duct infections. Aalasi's older sister had an eye infection when she was young. Ijisiuti was placed directly on her eyeball, left overnight, and covered with a cloth eye patch. Her eye soon healed.

ᐃᔾᓯᐅᑎ ᐊᑐᖅᑕᐅᔪᓐᓇᓂᕗᑦ, ᐃᔾᓄᒃᑐᓄᑦ. ᓂᑦᓕᓇᑦᑎᐊᖅᑐᐊᓘᕗᑦ ᐊᑲᐅᑦᑐᑎᑦᑐ ᐃᔾᒍᑦ ᐃᓕᔭᐅᑎᑦᑐᒋᑦ. ᐊᑐᖅᑕᐅᔪᓐᓇᖅᒥᔪᑦ ᐃᔾᔨᓯᒪᑐᐃᓐᓇᖅᑐᓄᑦ.

Ijisiuti can also be used to soothe sore red eyes. It is cool and refreshing when placed on the eyelids. It can also be used to help remove something from the eye.

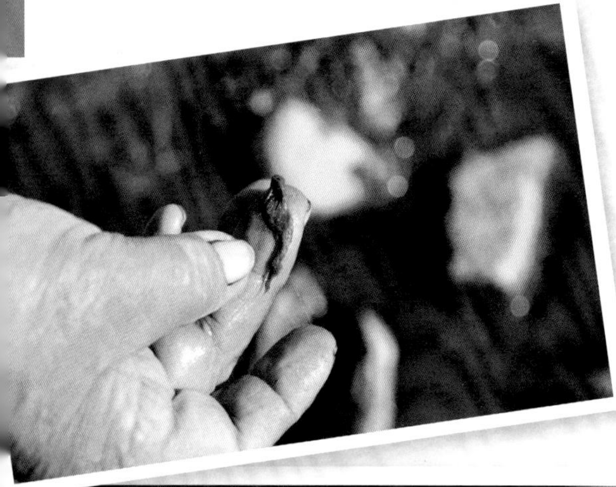

ᐊᑐᕐᓂᐊᕐᓗᒋᑦ ᐃᔨᓯᐅᑎ, ᐲᔭᕋᕈᕕᒋᑦ ᓴᓂᐅᑦᑕᐃᓕᑎᑦᑎᐊᕿᔭᖅᐸᑎᑦ (ᓯᐅᕿ ᐊᒻᒪ ᒪᕐᕿᕈᔫᖕᒋᑦᓗᑎᕐ). ᐃᔨᓯᐅᑎ ᓴᖖᒋᓂᖅᐹᖕᒍᕐᑲᑦᑕᖅᑐᑦ ᐋᒡᒌᓯᐅᑉ ᓄᖖᒍᐊᓂ ᐊᒻᒪ ᓯᑎᐱᕆᒥᑦ. ᐃᔨᓯᐅᑎᑦ ᑐᕐᑯᓕᖕᒐᖕᒋᑦᑎᐊᕐᓗᑎᒃ ᑭᓯᐊᓂ ᐊᑐᖁᒃᓴᐅᓂᖕᒋᓐᓄᑦ ᐊᐅᔭᒃᑯᑐᐊᖅ ᐊᑐᖅᑕᐅᓲᖕᒍᕗᑦ.

To use ijisiuti, make sure it is clean when you pull it out of the water (no sand or dirt). Choose darker green ijisiuti, as it is riper. Ijisiuti is most potent in late August and September. Ijisiuti should be used fresh from the water and therefore can only be used in the summer.

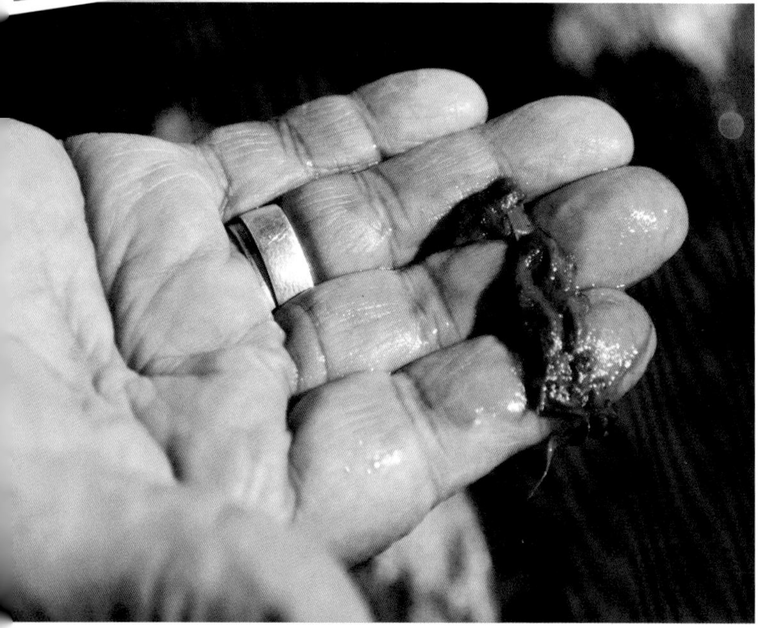

ᐃᔨᓯᐅᑎᑦ ᐊᑲᐅᓯᓴᐅᑎᐅᔪᓐᓇᖅᑐᑦ ᐃᔨᓗᒃᑐᓄᑦ, ᐊᒻᒪ ᐃᔨᐅᑉ ᑭᑦᓚᖕᒐᓄᑦ ᕐᑯᕝᕕᐅᕐᕕᓄᑦᓗ.

Ijisiuti can help with many ailments of the eye, including irritations of the skin around the eye and infections of the tear duct.

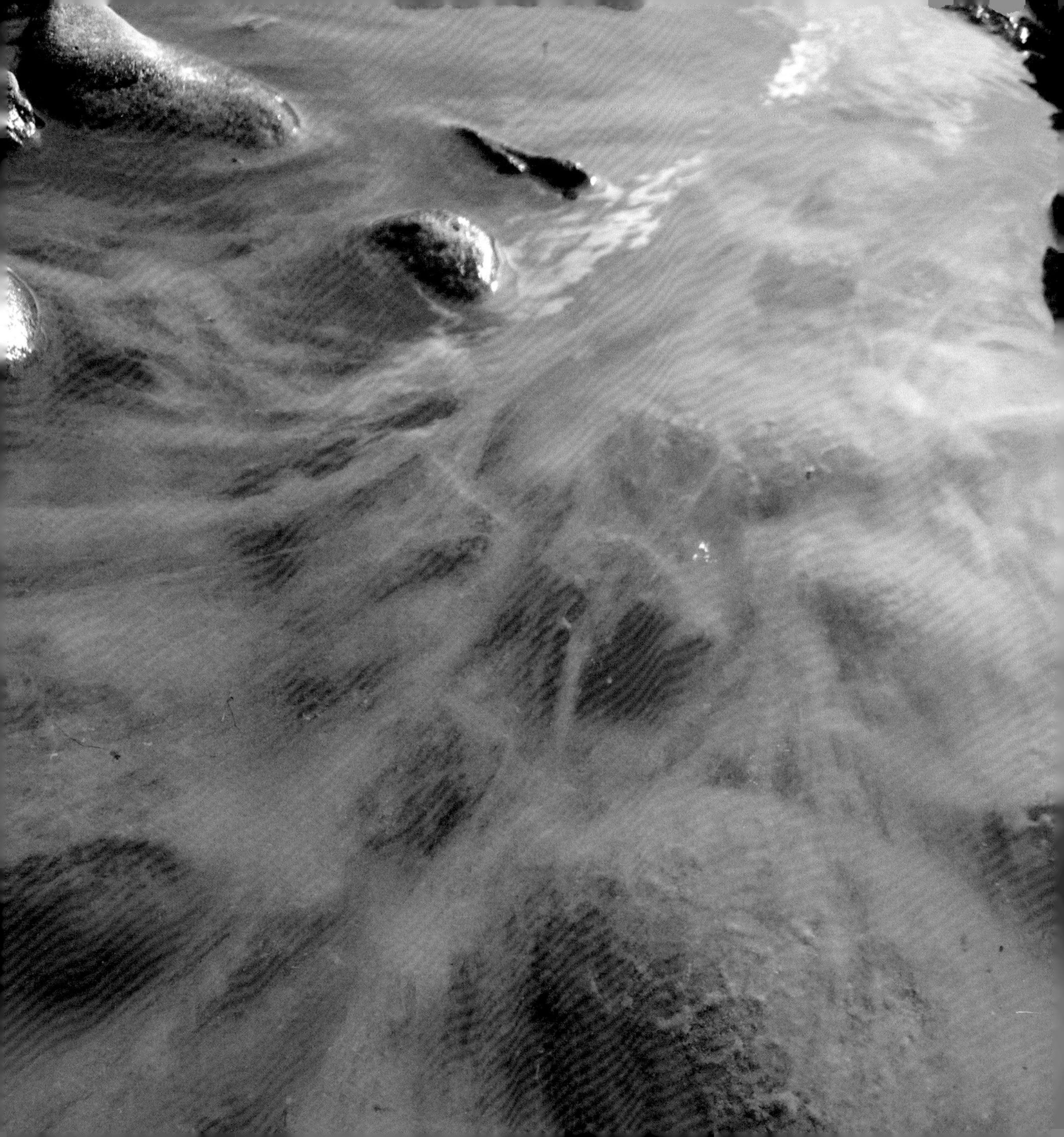

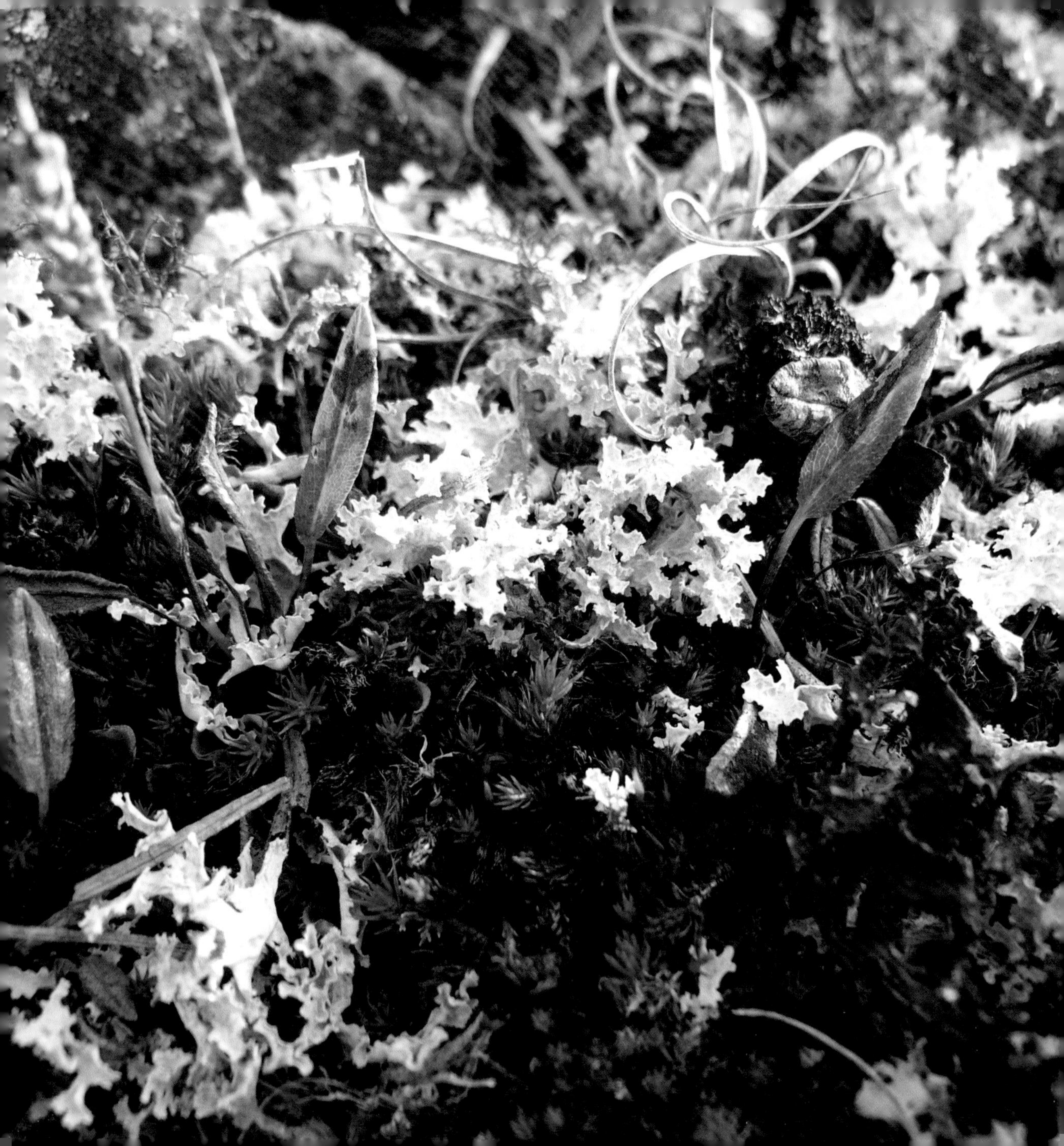

ᓂᕐᓇᐃᑦ
Nirnait / Snow Lichen

ᓂᕐᓇᐃᑦ ᓇᓂᔭᕐᓂᖅᑐᑯᓘᕗᑦ—ᖃᑯᖅᑕᑯᓗᐃᑦ ᓯᓂᖏᑦ ᐃᒧᓗᖅᑳᓯᒪᔪᑯᓗᐃᑦ ᑕᖅᓴᐅᑦᑎᐊᖃᑦᑕᖅᑐᑦ ᑐᖑᔪᖅᑕᓂᒃ ᐱᕈᖅᑐᓂᒃ ᐊᒻᒪᓗ ᐊᓯᖏᓐᓂᑦ ᐱᕈᖅᑐᓂᑦ ᓄᓇᔭᒥᑦ. ᓂᕐᓇᐃᑦ ᐊᑯᓂᐊᓗᒃ ᐱᕈᕋᓱᖃᑦᑕᖅᑐᑦ, ᓵᕐᓗ ᐊᓯᖏᑦ ᑐᒃᑐᓄᑦ ᓂᖀᑦ ᑕᐃᒪᐃᑉᐸᒻᒪᑕ. ᓱᕈᓯᐅᓪᓗᓂᑦ ᐋᓚᓯ ᐅᖃᐅᔾᔭᐅᖃᑦᑕᓚᐅᖅᓯᒪᔪᖅ ᓂᕐᓇᓂᑦ ᐊᓯᖏᓐᓂᓗ ᐱᕈᖅᑐᓂᑦ ᑐᓪᓕᕋᖃᑦᑕᖁᔭᐅᒐᓂ ᐊᑯᓂᐊᓗᒃ ᐱᕈᒃᑲᓐᓂᕋᓱᓲᖑᒻᒪᑕ. ᓂᕐᓇᐃᑦᑕᐅᖅ ᐱᒻᒪᕆᐅᕗᑦ ᑐᒃᑐᓄᑦ ᓂᕿᒋᔭᐅᒻᒪᑕ.

Nirnait (snow lichen) is easy to spot—its ivory fingers with crinkled edges stand out from soft green mosses and other plants on the tundra. Like other lichens, nirnait takes a long time to grow. As a child, Aalasi was told to avoid stepping on nirnait, and other plants, to show respect and because it takes so long to regenerate. Also, nirnait is an important food source for caribou.

ᓂᕐᓇᐃᑦ ᐊᑐᖅᑕᐅᔪᓐᓇᖅᑐᑦ ᐊᑲᐅᓯᓴᐅᑎᐅᓗᑎᒃ ᖃᓂᒪᓂᑦ ᐊᓂᐊᑦᑎᔪᓐᓇᕐᒪᑦ ᐊᐅᒪᔮᕐᓂᒃᑯᑦ. ᑏᖖᒍᐊᑦ ᓂᕐᓇᓂᑦ ᓴᓇᓯᒪᔪᖅ ᐊᐅᒪᔾᔭᒍᑕᐅᔪᓐᓇᕐᒪᑦ ᐃᓄᒻᒧᑦ. ᐋᓚᓯ ᐃᖅᑲᐅᒪᔪᖅ ᐊᓈᓇᖓ ᑏᖖᒍᐊᓕᐅᕈᔾᔨᓚᐅᖅᓯᒪᒻᒪᑦ ᖃᓂᒪᔪᒥᒃ ᐅᑭᐅᖑᑎᓪᓗᒍ. ᐋᓚᓯᐅᑉ ᐊᓈᓇᖓ ᐃᓪᒃᑯᐊᓂᑦ ᓂᕐᓇᓂᑦ ᐊᒥᐊᒃᑯᓯᒪᓐᓂᕐᒪᑦ ᐅᑭᐅᖑᑎᓪᓗᒍ. ᑏᖖᒍᐊᖅ ᐃᒥᓚᐅᖅᑐᓂᐅᑉ, ᐊᑯᓂᐅᖏᑦᑐᖅ ᐊᑲᐅᓯᔪᕙᓂᖅ ᑕᐃᓐᓇ ᐃᓄᒃ. ᐊᓯᒃᑲᓐᓂᐊᒍᑦ ᐋᓚᓯ ᐅᑭᐅᖃᖅᑐᓂ 24ᐸᓗᖕᓂᑦ ᖃᑕᖖᒍᑎᒌᑦ ᖃᓂᒪᓕᓚᐅᖅᓯᒪᓐᓂᕐᒪᑕ, ᐊᑕᖏᖅᑐᑎᒃ ᖃᓂᒪᖏᑦᑐᑑᓕᖅᑐᓂ. ᐃᖅᑲᐅᒪᒐᒥᑦ ᐊᑲᐅᓯᔾᔭᑕᐅᔭᓇᕐᓂᖏᑦ ᓂᕐᓇᐃᑦ, ᑏᖖᒍᐊᓕᐅᕈᑎᓚᐅᖅᓯᒪᔭᕙᓂᖏᑦ ᓂᕐᓇᓂᒃ ᐃᓚᓂ. ᐃᑲᕐᕋᐅᑉ ᐊᖕᖏᓪᓗᐊᖓ ᐊᓂᒍᖅᓯᒪᓕᖅᑎᓪᓗᒍ ᐃᓚᖏᑦ ᐊᐅᒪᔮᖅᑐᐊᓘᓕᖅᑐᕙᓃᑦ. ᐃᓚᖏᑕ ᐃᓚᖏᑦ ᕿᑲᑐᐃᓐᓇᕈᓐᓃᖅᑐᕙᓃᑦ, ᐃᓚᖏᓪᓗ ᖃᐅᑐᐃᓐᓇᖅᑎᓪᓗᒍ ᐊᑲᐅᓯᓕᓪᓗᑎᑦ.

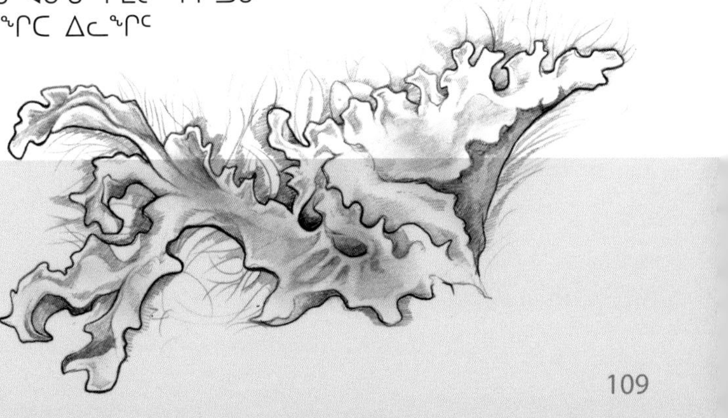

Nirnait can be used as a medicine for illnesses that need to be sweated out. Nirnait tea causes a person to sweat. Aalasi recalls that her mother once made nirnait tea for someone who was sick in the winter. Aalasi's mother had saved a small parcel of nirnait for the winter. Soon after drinking the tea, the person became better. Another time, when Aalasi was about twenty-four years old, her entire family became very sick except for her. She remembered the healing properties of nirnait, so she served her family nirnait tea. About half an hour after drinking the nirnait tea, they began to sweat profusely. Some of them became active the following day and the others were feeling better soon after.

ᓂᕐᓇᐃᑦ ᓂᕆᔭᐅᔭᕆᐊᖅᑲᙱᓚᖅ. ᑏᙳᐊᓕᐊᕆᓗᒍ ᑭᓯᐊᓂ ᐱᐅᒪᑕ. ᓂᕐᓇᓂᒃ ᑏᙳᐊᓕᐅᕐᓂᐊᕈᕕᑦ, ᑎᖅᑎᑎᑲᐃᓐᓇᖅᑐᐃᓐᓇᕐᓗᒍ ᓈᒻᒪᒃᑲᔭᖅᑐᖅ, ᐃᓱᖅᓯᓇᓱᑐᐃᓐᓇᕐᓂᙵᓂᑦ. ᐃᒥᕐᓂᐊᖅᑐᐃᓐᓇᕐᓗᒍ ᑎᓴᐃᖓᓕᖅᐸᑦ. ᓂᕐᓇᐃᑦ ᖃᔅᔫᓐᓇᒍᓗᐃᑦ ᑏᓕᐅᕈᑎᒥᑦ ᑕᑕᐃᕙᓐᓇᖅᐳᑦ. ᐊᒻᒪᓗ ᐃᕐᖑᓯᖅ ᐊᑕᐅᓯᖅ ᓈᒻᒪᑐᐃᓐᓇᖅᑐᓂ. ᓂᕐᓇᐃᑦ ᑏᙳᐊᖑᑦᑐᓗᒍ ᓴᙱᕙᑭᔫᒻᒪᑦ, ᓄᑕᕋᕐᓄ ᐱᔭᐅᔭᕆᐊᖅᑲᙱᑦᑐᖅ. ᓂᕐᓇᐃᑦ ᖃᙵᑐᐃᓐᓇᑦᑎᐊᖅ ᓄᐊᑕᒃᓴᐅᕗᑦ, ᑭᓯᐊᓂᓕ ᐴᖅᓯᒪᓗᒥᑦ ᖃᐅᒪᔪᑭᓵᒥᑦ ᐱᐅᑦᑎᐊᖅᑐᑦ. ᓂᕐᓇᐃᑦ ᓂᑲᒋᔭᐅᔭᕆᐊᖅᑲᖅᑐᑦ, ᖃᑦᑐᓈᖅᑕᒦᑦᑐᑎᒃ, ᐊᑭᓯᐅᑦᓘᓐᓃᑦ ᐴᖓᓂᑦ ᓂᑦᓚᓯᑦᑐᒦᑦᑐᑏᑦ.

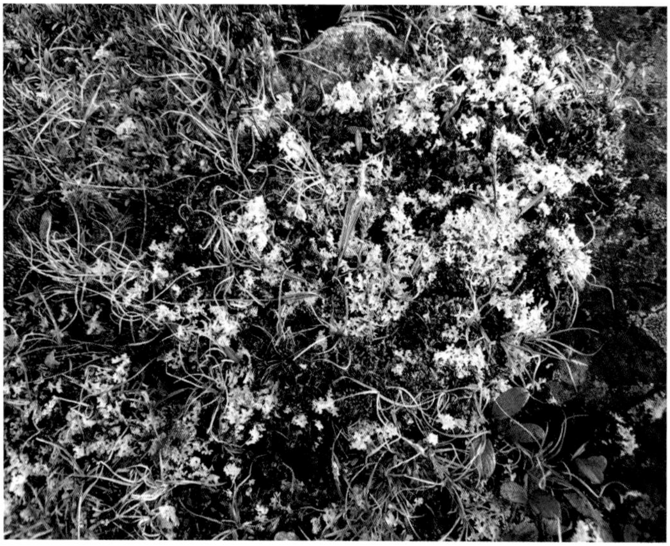

ᓂᕐᓇᐃᑦ ᐃᒧᑭᔫᔭᖅᓯᒪᔪᑯᓗᐃᑦ ᑕᖅᓴᐅᑦᑎᐊᖅᑐᑦ, ᓲᕐᓗᑕ ᐊᐳᑎ ᓄᓇᔭᒥᑦ.

The bright, crinkled fingers of nirnait resemble a patch of snow on the tundra.

Nirnait should not be eaten. It should only be consumed as a tea. To make nirnait tea, simply boil the nirnait briefly, until the water becomes dark. Drink it when it has cooled. Only a small handful of nirnait is needed to make a pot of tea, and one cup of the tea is enough to be effective. Because nirnait tea is so powerful, it probably should not be given to babies. Nirnait can be collected at any time, but it is best not to store it in plastic. It should be handled gently and stored in a flour sack, some canvas, or in something like a pillowcase.

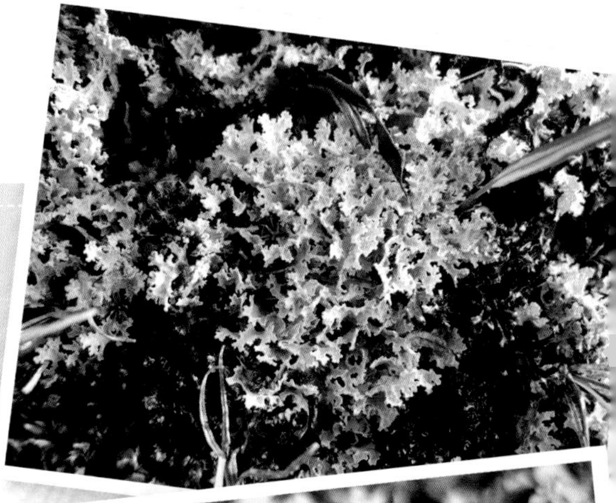

ᓂᕐᓇᐃᑦ ᐊᑯᓂᐊᓗᒃ ᐱᕈᕋᓱᓲᑦ. ᐋᓚᓯᓕ ᐃᖅᑲᐅᒪᕗᖅ ᑐᓪᓕᕋᖅᑲᑦᑕᕐᑯᔭᐅᑎᓐᓇᒋᑦ ᐱᔫᓇᓗᓂᑦ.

Nirnait takes a long time to grow, so Aalasi was always told to avoid stepping on it, she recalls.

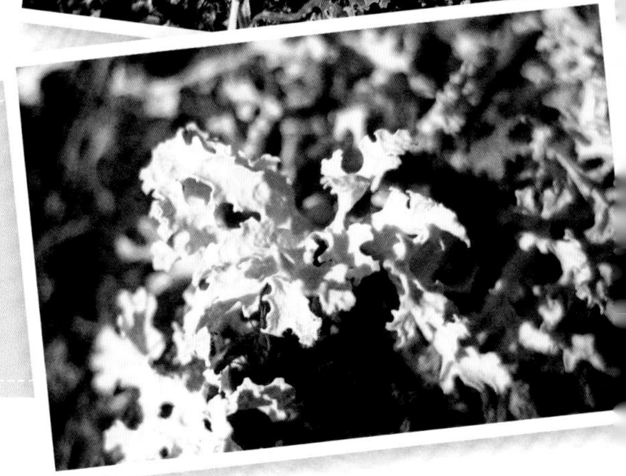

ᓂᕐᓇᐃᑦ ᕐᑲᑯᑦᑎᐊᖅᑐᐊᓘᕐᑲᑦᑕᖅᑐᑦ ᓯᕐᑭᓂᖅ ᓂᐱᓕᖅᑎᓪᓗᒍ.

Nirnait appears ivory coloured in the low light of dusk.

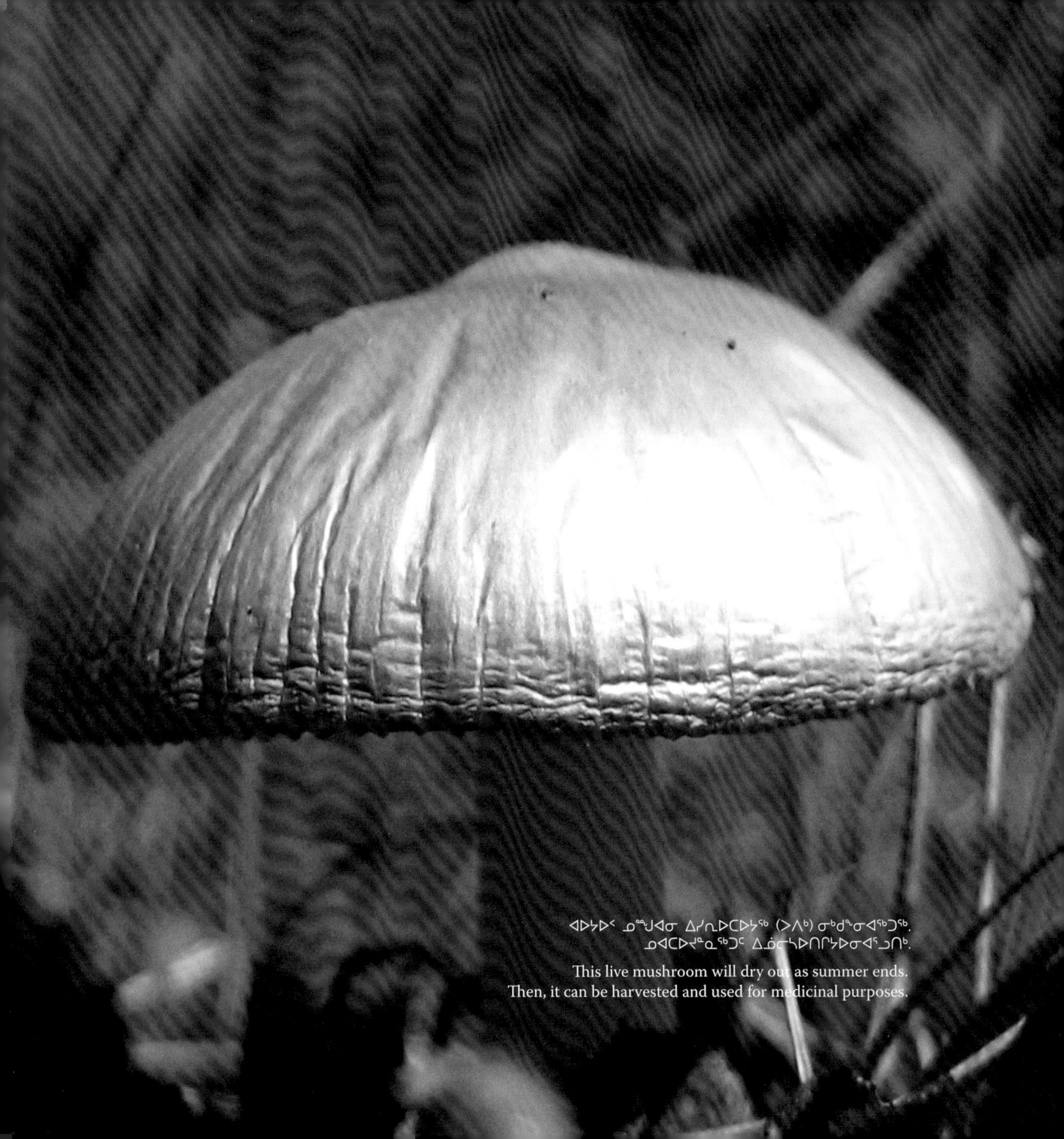

ᐊᐅᔭᐅᑉ ᓄᙳᐊᓂ ᐃᓯᓇᐅᑕᐅᔭᖅ (ᐳᐱᒃ) ᓂᒃᑯᖕᓂᐊᖅᑐᖅ.
ᓄᐊᑕᐅᔪᓐᓇᖅᑐᑦ ᐃᓘᓕᔭᐅᑎᒋᔭᐅᓂᐊᕐᓗᑎᒃ.

This live mushroom will dry out as summer ends.
Then, it can be harvested and used for medicinal purposes.

ᐳᔪᐊᓗᒃ
Pujualuk / Dried Mushroom

ᐳᔪᐊᓗᒃ (ᐸᓂᖅᓯᒪᔪᖅ ᐃᓯᓇᐅᑕᐅᔭᖅ) ᓇᓂᔭᕐᓂᖏᑦᑐᑦ ᓵᖅᑲᐃᒻᒪ ᑕᖅᓴᐅᖏᑦᑐᑯᓗᐃᑦ ᖁᖅᓯᐸᓗᒃᑐᑎᒃ ᑲᔪᐃᑦ ᑕᕐᕋᓕᓂᕐᒦᒡᒍᔪᐊᓘᓪᓗᑎᓪᓗ ᐱᕈᖅᑐᐃᑦ ᑕᑭᔪᐃᑦ ᐅᖕᖓᓘᓐᓃᑦ ᐅᔭᕋᐃᑦ ᓴᓂᕋᖏᓐᓂ. ᐳᔪᐊᓗᒃᓯᐅᕐᓂᐊᕈᕕᑦ, ᕿᓂᓇᐊᖅᑲᖅᑐᑎᑦ ᓯᐅᕌᔭᒥᐅᖏᑦᑐᖅ, ᓄᓇᔭᒥ ᑭᓯᐊᓂ.

It is not easy to spot a *pujualuk* (dried mushroom) because they are generally dull beige in colour, and they tend to appear in the shadows of taller plants and rocks. To find a pujualuk, look in areas without gravel, where the soil is richer.

ᐳᔪᐊᓗᒃ ᐋᑎᓕᒻᒪᕇᑦ ᒪᑦᑐᑎᑦᑎᐊᕚᓘᑦᓗᑎᓪᓗ. ᓯᕈᔾᔨᒃᑯᑎᑦᑎᐊᕚᓗᐃᑦ ᐊᒻᒪᓗ ᐊᐅᓈᖅᑐᒥᑦ ᓯᒥᑦᑐᐃᑦᑎᐊᖅᑐᑎᒃ. ᐳᔪᐊᓗᒃ ᐊᒥᕐᓗᕈᔭᓂᒃ ᐱᐅᓯᕚᑦᑕᖅᑎᑦᑎᔭᓇᑦᑎᐊᕐᒥᔪᑦ, ᓵᕐᓗ ᐅᕕᓂᕐᓗᖕᓂᑦ ᐊᒻᒪᓗ ᐊᓯᕈᓘᔭᖏᓐᓂᑦ. ᐳᔪᐊᓗᓐᓂᒃ ᐊᑐᕐᓂᐊᕐᓗᓂ, ᑭᑦᑕᓚᑦ ᐅᖕᖓᓘᓐᓃᑦ ᐊᒥᕐᓗᓚᑦ ᓱᖁᑐᐃᓐᓇᕐᓗᒍ ᐃᑕᔪᓐᓇᖅᑕᐃᑦ ᐳᔪᕈᔫᓂᖓ ᐅᕕᓂᖕᖓᑦ ᐊᑦᑐᐊᖕᒑᕐᓗᓂ. ᖃᐅᔨᒪᔭᐅᔭᓇᐊᓕᒃ:

A pujualuk can be very useful as a bandage. It will protect the wound, and it contains vital blood-clotting chemicals that can help to stop bleeding. A pujualuk can also alleviate general skin problems, such as rashes and other irritations. To use a pujualuk, simply break it open and place it, powdery side down, on the wound or skin irritation.

ᐳᔪᐊᓗᒃ ᐸᓂᖅᓯᒪᔪᖅ ᑭᓯᐊᓂ ᐱᐅᒐᖅ ᐸᓂᖅᓯᒪᖏᒃᑯᓂ ᐊᑲᐅᓯᓴᐅᑎᖅᑲᖏᒻᒪᑦ.

Note: live mushrooms do not have the medicinal properties that dried mushrooms have.

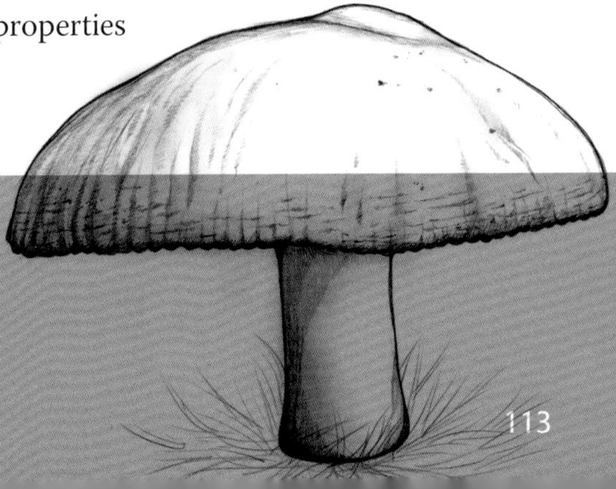

ᐳᔪᐊᓗᒃ ᐊᐅᔭᓕᒫᖅ ᓄᐊᑕᒃᓴᑦ ᐊᒻᒪ ᐃᓕᒃᑯᐊᕆᔭᒃᓴᐅᔪᑦ ᐱᐅᔪᓐᓃᕈᓐᓇᖏᑦ. ᐋᓚᓯ ᐃᖅᑲᐅᒪᔪᖅ ᐊᓈᓇᖓ ᐴᖅᓯᒪᔪᓂᒃ ᐳᔪᐊᓗᖃᐃᓐᓇᖅᑕᓚᐅᖅᓯᒪᒻᒪᑦ ᑭᓕᖅᑐᖃᓂᕈᓂ ᓇᑦᓕᐅᒃᑯᒫᕆᑦᑐᓂᒋᑦ. ᐊᕕᙵᐃᑦ ᐊᒥᕕᓂᖏᓐᓂᑦ ᐴᖅᑲᖅᑎᖢᒐᖅᑕᓚᐅᖅᓯᒪᔭᖏᑦ ᐱᔾᔪᑎᒋᓪᓗᒍ ᐊᕕᙵᐃᑦ ᐊᒥᖏᑦ ᓂᕈᒥᒃᑐᑰᒻᒪᑕ ᓱᕿᑎᕆᖏᒻᒪᑕ ᓂᑲᓇᖅᑐᓂᑦ ᐳᔪᐊᓗᓐᓂᑦ. ᐳᔪᐊᓗᓐᓂᑦ ᐱᓂᐊᕈᕕᑦ ᖄᖓ ᓯᕿᑦᑕᐃᓕᒪᑦᑎᐊᕐᓗᒍ ᐳᔪᐋᓂᖓ ᔭᖁᑐᐃᓐᓇᑦᑕᕐᓂᐊᕐᒪᑦ.

A pujualuk can be collected during the summer months and stored indefinitely. Aalasi recalls that her mother always kept a pouch of them handy just in case someone was injured. She preferred to store them in a lemming pelt bag because the padding and softness of the lemming pelt would protect the fragile pujualuk. When picking a pujualuk, try not to rupture the outer skin any more than necessary so that the powdery insides stay intact.

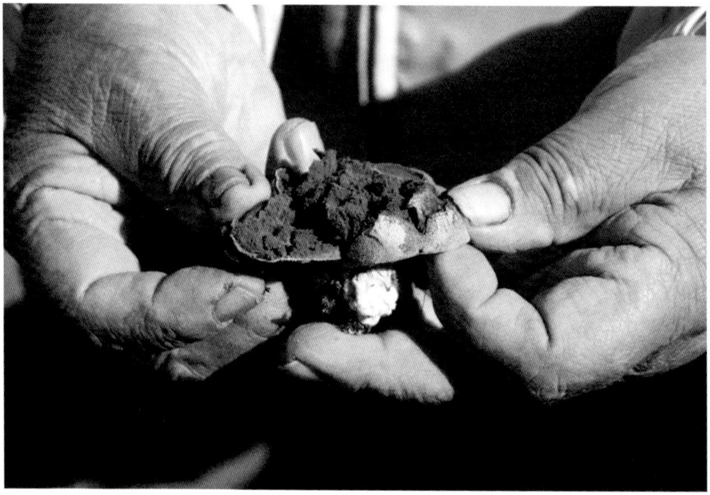

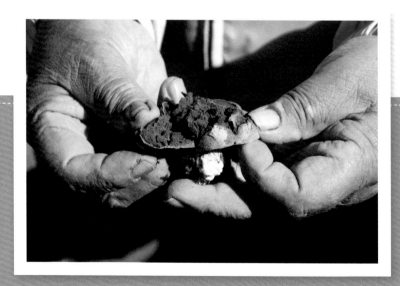

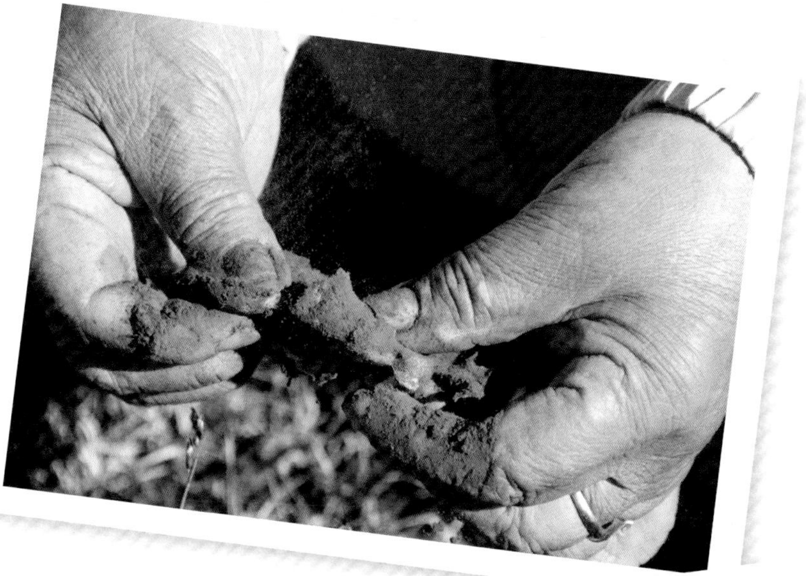

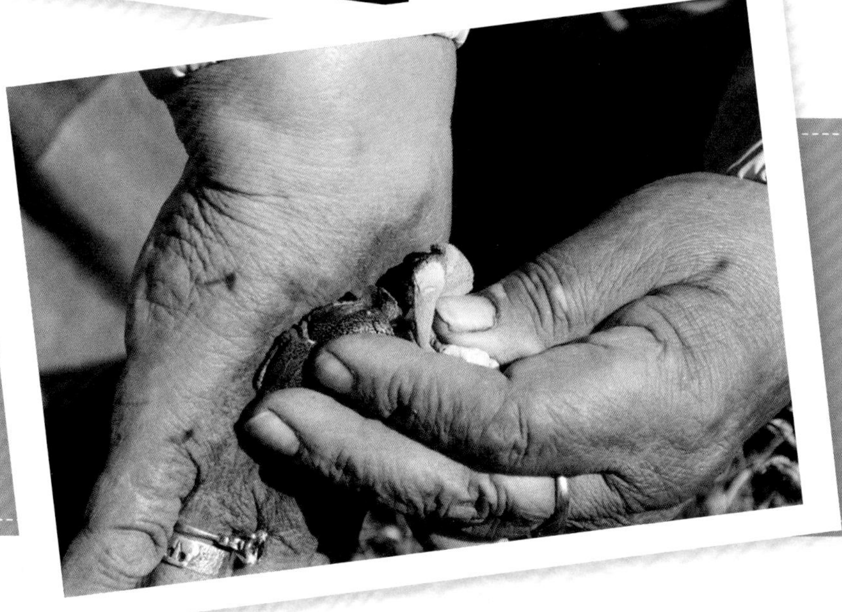

ᐋᓚᓯ ᐳᔪᐊᓗᒻᒥᑦ
ᒪᑉᐱᖅᓯᔪᖅ
ᖄᓇᖅ ᑭᑦᑕᓇᑦ
ᐊᑐᖅᑕᐅᓲᖑᒻᒪᖓᑕ
ᑕᑯᑎᑦᑎᓂᐊᕐᒥᒃ.

Aalasi opens a
powdery pujualuk
and demonstrates
how she would
place it on a wound.

ᐊᑐᒪᒃᓴᒃᑲᓐᓃᑦ
Additional Resources

ᑐᑭᓯᒋᐊᒃᑲᓐᓂᕈᒪᒍᕕᑦ ᐱᕈᖅᑐᐃᑦ ᐅᖃᓕᒫᒐᕐᒦᑦᑐᑦ ᒥᒃᓵᓄᑦ, ᐅᑯᐊ ᐊᑐᕈᒪᑐᐃᓐᓇᕆᐊᓕᒃᑎᑦ.

If you would like more information about the plants in this book, you may want to use the following resources.

- ᓄᓇᕗᒻᒥ ᐱᕈᖅᑐᐃᑦ. 2013 (revised edition). ᑭᐅᕈᓚᓐ ᒫᓗᕆ, ᓲᓴᓐ ᐊᐃᑲᓐ. ᓄᓇᕗᑦ ᐃᓕᓐᓂᐊᖅᑐᓕᕆᔨᒃᑯᑦ, ᐃᖃᓗᐃᑦ, ᓄᓇᕗᑦ. (ᖃᓪᓗᓈᑎᑐᑦ ᐃᓄᒃᑎᑐᓪᓗ)

  Common Plants of Nunavut. 2013 (revised edition). Carolyn Mallory and Susan Aiken. Inhabit Media, Iqaluit, Nunavut. (English)

- ᓄᓇᔭᒥᑦ ᐱᐅᔪᐃᑦ: ᐱᕕᐊᕐᓇᖅᑐᑦ ᓄᓇᕋᐃᑦ ᑲᓇᑕᐅᑉ ᐅᑭᐅᖅᑕᖅᑐᖓᓂᑦ. 2004 (ᓴᓇᔭᐅᕆᐊᒃᑲᓐᓂᖅᓯᒪᔪᑦ). ᐸᐃᔾ ᕘᑦ. ᐊᑉ ᕼᐃᐅ ᓴᖅᑭᑎᑦᑎᔩᑦ, ᔭᓗᓇᐃᕝ, ᓄᓇᑦᓯᐊᖅ. (ᖃᓪᓗᓈᑎᑐᑦ ᐊᒻᒪᓗ ᓇᐃᓪᓕᑎᖅᓯᒪᔭᓖᑦ ᐃᓄᐃᓐᓇᖅᑐᑦ)

  Barrenland Beauties: Showy Plants of the Canadian Arctic. 2004 (revised edition). Page Burt. Uphere Publishing, Yellowknife, Northwest Territories. (English with summaries in Inuinnaqtun)

- ᖃᐅᔨᓇᓱᒌᑎᑦ ᐊᑯᓐᓂᑦᑎᓐᓂᑦ ᐅᑭᐅᖅᑕᖅᑐᒥ. 1994. ᐃ.ᓯ. ᐸᐃᓗ. ᓯᓚᑦᑐᖅᓴᕐᕕᔾᔪᐊᒥᑦ ᓰᑲᒍ ᐳᕋᔅ, ᓰᑲᒍ, ᐃᓕᓄᐃ. (ᖃᓪᓘᓈᑎᑑᖅᑐᑦ)

  A Naturalist's Guide to the Arctic. 1994. E. C. Pielou. The University of Chicago Press, Chicago, Illinois. (English only)

- ᐊᐱᖅᓱᕐᓂᖅ ᐃᓄᐃᑦ ᐃᓐᓇᕐᓂᓐᓂᑦ: ᖃᓄᐃᑦᑕᐃᓕᒪᓇᓲᑎᑐᖃᐃᑦ ᑎᒥᒧᑦ. 2001. ᐃᓕᓴᐱ ᐆᑦᑐᕗ, ᑎᐹᓚ ᖃᐱᒃ ᐊᑕᒍᑦᓯᐊᖅ, ᑎᑎᓯ ᐃᔾᔭᖏᐊᖅ, ᔭᐃᑯ ᐱᑦᓯᐅᓚᒃ, ᐋᓚᓯ ᔫᒥ, ᐊᑭᓱ ᔫᒥ, ᒪᓚᐃᔭ ᐸᐹᑦᓯ. ᐋᖅᑭᒋᐊᖅᓱᐳ ᒥᓯᐅᑦ ᑐᕆᐃᓐ ᐊᒻᒪ ᕗᕆᑦᑐᕆᒃ ᓚᒍᕋᑦ. ᓄᓇᕗᑦ ᓯᓚᑦᑐᖅᓴᕐᕕᒃ, ᐃᖃᓗᐃᑦ, ᓄᓇᕗᑦ. (ᖃᑦᔭᓈᑎᑐᑦ ᐃᓄᒃᑎᑐᓪᓗ)

  Interviewing Inuit Elders: Perspectives on Traditional Health. 2001. Ilisapi Ootoova, Tipuula Qaapik Atagutsiak, Tirisi Ijjangiaq, Jaikku Pitseolak, Aalasi Joamie, Akisu Joamie, and Malaija Papatsie. Edited by Michèle Therrien and Frédéric Laugrand. Nunavut Arctic College, Iqaluit, Nunavut. (English and Inuktitut)

- ᐊᑲᐅᓯᓴᐅᑎᑐᖃᓕᕆᓂᖅ: ᐅᓂᒃᑳᓕᐊᖑᓯᒪᔪᑦ, *ᓰᑎᐱᕆ 28, 1983*. 1984. ᔫᓇᑕᓂ ᓯᑏᕗ. ᐊᕗᑕ ᐃᓕᖅᑯᓯᓕᕆᓂᖅ, ᐃᓄᒃᔪᐊᖅ, ᑯᐸᐃᒃ. (ᖃᑦᔭᓈᑎᑐᑦ ᐃᓄᒃᑎᑐᓪᓗ)

  Traditional Medicine Project: Interim Report, September 28, 1983. 1984. Jonathan Stevens. Avataq Cultural Institute, Inukjuaq, Quebec. (English and Inuktitut)

ᑎᑎᕋᖅᑐᕕᓃᑦ
Contributors

ᐋᓚᓯ ᔮᒥ ᐃᓅᓂᑯ ᐃᓄᒃᔪᐊ, ᑯᐸᐃᒻᒥᑦ. ᖃᑕᙳᑎᖏᑦ ᓄᑦᑎᕐᓂᑯᐃᑦ ᐸᓐᓂᖅᑑᒧᑦ ᓂᕕᐊᖅᓯᐊᙳᑎᓪᓗᒍ. 1960ᒥᑦ, ᓄᑦᑎᕐᓂᑯ ᐅᐃᒦᑦ ᕿᑐᙵᓃᑦ ᓂᐊᖁᙶᒧᑦ ᐃᓪᓗᑖᕆᐅᖅᑐᑎᓪᓗ. ᑕᐃᒪᙵᓂ ᓂᐊᖁᙶᒥᐅᑕᐅᔪᖅ. ᐊᖀᒍᒐᓚᖕᓂᑦ, ᓇᔾᔨᔭᑕᕆᔨᐅᖅᑲᑕᐅᓚᐅᖅᓯᒪᔭᖅ ᐋᓂᐊᕕᒻᒥᑦ. ᐋᓚᓯ ᐊᐱᖅᓱᖅᑕᐅᖅᑕᐅᓂᑰᒻᒥᔭᖅ ᐃᓐᓇᕐᓂᑦ ᐅᖃᓕᒫᒐᕐᒧᑦ ᖃᓄᐃᑦᑕᐃᓕᒪᔾᔭᑎᑐᖃᐃᑦ ᑎᒥᒧᑦ ᐊᒻᒪ ᐃᓕᓐᓂᐊᖅᑎᑎᓲᖑᓪᓗᓂ ᐱᕈᖅᑐᑦ ᒥᒃᓵᓄᑦ ᓯᓚᑦᑐᖅᓴᕕᒻᒥᑦ. ᐊᐅᓪᓚᖅᑕᐅᕙᑦᑐᓂᓗ ᑲᓇᑕᒥ ᓯᓚᑖᓄᑦ ᐱᕈᖅᑐᑦ ᐊᑑᑎᖏᑦ ᐅᓂᒃᑳᕆᔭᖅᑐᖅᑐᒥᑦ.

Aalasi Joamie was born in Inukjuak, Quebec. Her family moved to Pangnirtung when she was a young girl. In the 1960s, she moved to Niaqunnguuq (Apex) with her husband and children into their first house. She has lived there ever since. For many years, Aalasi worked as a maternity aid at Baffin Regional Hospital. Aalasi contributed to *Interviewing Inuit Elders: Perspectives on Traditional Health* and she teaches traditional plant knowledge workshops at Nunavut Arctic College. She also travels to traditional plant-use conferences nationally and internationally.

ᐋᓇ ᓯᒡᓗᕐ ᖁᑦᑎᖕᓂᖅᐸᐅᒐᖅ ᐅᑭᐅᖅᑕᖅᑐᒥ ᓱᐳᑏᑦ ᖃᐅᔨᓇᓱᐊᖅᑎᒃᑯᓐᓂᑦ, ᐱᑕᕆᑦᑐᐊᑕᓲᑦ ᐱᕚᓪᓕᐊᓂᕐᒥᒃ ᖃᐅᔨᓴᕐᓂᕐᒥᒃ ᓄᓇᓕᖕᓂ ᖃᓄᐃᖕᒋᑦᑎᐊᕋᓱᐊᕐᓂᕐᒥ, ᐊᔪᖅᓴᖅᑕᐃᓕᒪᑎᑦᑎᓂᕐᒥᒃ, ᐃᓐᓇᕐᓂᓪᓗ ᐃᓕᓐᓂᐊᖅᑐᓂᒃ. ᐱᑕᕆᐊᖅᑲᓚᐅᖅᓯᒪᑎᓪᓗᒍ ᓯᕗᓪᓕᖅᐹᒥ ᐱᓱᖅᑎᖅᑲᕐᓂᖅ ᐋᓚᓯᒥ, ᐱᔭᕇᖅᓯᐊᕕᓂᖅ ᖃᐅᔨᓴᕐᓂᕐᒥᒃ ᑐᖅᑯᖅᑐᐃᓂᕐᒥᒃ ᐃᓄᐃᑦ ᖃᐅᔨᒪᔭᙱᓐᓂᒃ. ᐃᖃᓗᖕᒥᐅᑕᐅᓚᐅᖅᓯᒪᑎᓪᓗᒍ ᓄᓇᕗᒻᒥ, ᐊᖀᒍᓂᒃ ᖁᓕᑦ ᓯᑕᒪᓪᓗ, ᐋᑐᕚᒥᐅᑕᐅᓕᖅᑐᖅ, ᐋᓐᑎᐅᕆᔭᒥ, ᐱᑕᕆᖅᑎᖅᑲᓲᙳᑦᑐᓂ ᑲᑎᙵᒐᔭᓂᒃ ᐃᓄᐃᑦ ᓄᓇᖓᓂ. ᑎᑎᕋᖅᑎᖅᑲᖅᓯᒪᒋᕗᖅ, ᕇᐱᑲ ᕼᐊᐃᓐᓄᒥ, ᓱᕈᓯᖅᓯᐅᒻᒥᒃ ᐊᔾᔨᙳᐊᓕᖕᒥᒃ ᐅᖃᓕᒫᒐᕐᒥᒃ ᐱᓱᖕᓂᖅ ᓄᓇᒃᑯᑦ, ᐃᓕᓴᐃᔭᖅ ᒪᒃᑯᒃᑐᓂᒃ ᐃᓅᓕᓴᐅᑎᐅᓲᓂᒃ ᓂᕆᔭᐅᓲᓂᒡᓗ ᐅᑭᐅᖅᑕᖅᑐᒥ ᐱᓱᖅᑐᓂᒃ.

Anna Ziegler is the principal of Arctic Willow Consulting, which specializes in program development and evaluation in community wellness, poverty reduction, and adult learning. Since working on the first edition of *Walking with Aalasi*, she has completed graduate research on practices of archiving Inuit traditional knowledge. After living in Iqaluit, Nunavut, for fourteen years, she now resides in Ottawa, Ontario, and works on projects with groups across Inuit Nunangat. She is also the co-author, with Rebecca Hainnu, of the children's picture book *A Walk on the Tundra,* which teaches young readers about medicinal and edible Arctic plants.

ᕇᐱᑲ ᕼᐊᐃᓐᓄ, ᑲᖏᖅᑐᒫᐱᒻᒥᐅᑕᖅ, ᓄᓇᕗᒻᒥ, ᐸᓂᖏᑦᑐ, ᑲᐃᑦᓕᓐ ᐊᒻᒪ ᓂᑮᑕ. ᐅᑉᐱᕆᔭᓕᒃ ᐃᓕᓐᓂᐊᖅᑎᑦᑎᓂᕐᒥᒃ ᐃᓄᐃᑦ ᖃᐅᔨᒪᔭᑐᖃᖏᓐᓂᑦ ᓄᓇᓂᒃ, ᐆᒪᔪᕐᓂᒃ, ᐃᓄᐃᑦ ᐊᑐᓚᐅᖅᑕᕕᓂᖏᓐᓂᒃ, ᐅᑉᐱᕈᓲᓯᖏᓐᓂᓪᓗ. ᐃᓚᒌᑦ ᖃᖓᑕᒫᒃᑯᑦ ᐊᐅᓪᓚᖅᓯᒪᒐᔪᑦᑐᑦ. ᖃᐅᔨᒪᔭᖏᓐᓂᒃ ᑎᑎᕋᕐᓂᕐᒥᑎᒍᑦ ᐃᓕᑕᐅᕐᑯᔨᕙᖅ. ᐱᓕᕆᐊᕆᓯᒪᔭᖏᑕ ᐃᓚᖏᑦ ᐃᒪᐅᑉ ᑕᕐᓂᖓᑦ, ᐱᑯᖕᓂᖅ ᓄᓇᒃᑯᑦ, ᓇᔪᓇᐃᔭᐃᓂᖅ ᕿᒥᕐᕈᓕᓐᓂᑦ. 2016 ᖑᑎᑦᑐᒍᑦ ᓵᓚᖃᐅᓯᐊᖅᑐᕕᓂᖅ ᐃᓕᓴᐃᔩᑦ ᑲᑐᔾᔨᖃᑎᒌᖏᓐᓂᑦ ᐃᓕᓴᐃᑎᐊᕐᓂᕐᒧᑦ.

Rebecca Hainnu lives in Clyde River, Nunavut, with her daughters, Katelyn and Nikita. Rebecca believes it is important to teach Inuit traditional knowledge about the land, animals, people, history, and philosophies. Her family is usually on the land throughout the seasons. She hopes to pass on some knowledge through her writing. Her work includes *The Spirit of the Sea, A Walk on the Tundra, A Walk on the Shoreline, Math Activities for Nunavut Classrooms,* and *Classifying Vertebrates.* Rebecca is an educator in a K–12 school. She was the recipient of the 2016 NTA Award for Teaching Excellence.

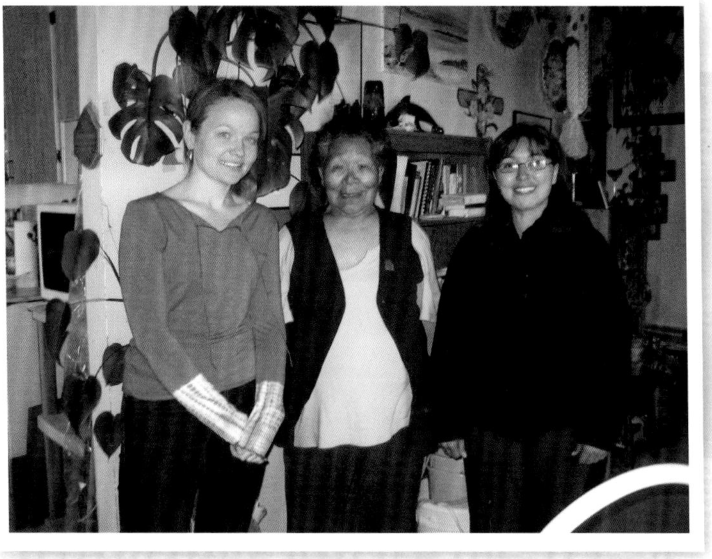

INHABIT MEDIA
Iqaluit • Toronto